Living the BONES Lifestyle

A Practical Guide To Conquering
The Fear Of Osteoporosis

Living the BONES Lifestyle

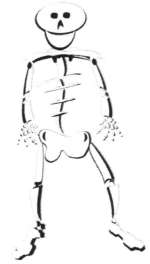

A Practical Guide To Conquering The Fear Of Osteoporosis

by
Cindy Killip

www.boneslifestyle.com

This publication is written and published to provide accurate and authoritative information relevant to the subject matter covered. It is published and sold with the understanding that neither the author nor publisher is engaged in rendering medical, psychological, financial, legal, or other professional services. If expert assistance or counseling is needed, the services of a competent professional should be sought.

Illustrations: ©Cindy Killip
Cover Photography: ©Laura Killip
Interior Eiffel Tower Photography: ©Kathy Dixon

Library of Congress Cataloging-in-Publication Data

Killip, Cindy
Living the BONES Lifestyle: A Practical Guide To Conquering The Fear Of Osteoporosis / Cindy Killip — 1st ed.
p. cm.
Includes bibliographical references and index
1. Health and Fitness—Exercise   2. Osteoporosis—Popular works.

ISBN-10: 1468050699
ISBN-13: 978-1468050691

Dedication

When your family believes in you and encourages your dreams, you can accomplish anything.

I dedicate this book to my family, especially my husband, Scott. He believed in me when I got overwhelmed, he guided me through the project's management, he taught me new technologies. He supported me through it all. This book marks another step in our journey together.

My children loved and encouraged me daily, provided much-needed breaks with their performances and sporting events, and rarely complained when dinner wasn't ready. My parents provided immeasurable support emotionally, physically, and financially not only with this project but throughout my life.

Thank you all.

Contents

Chapter 7
Exercise   103

Treasures

There is a Chinese Proverb that says, "Learning is a treasure that will follow its owner everywhere." That is my goal with this book, to give you a treasure. I want you to understand this thing called osteoporosis, so fear will no longer drive you but knowledge and courage will inspire you to take action. There are many people who have helped me bring this treasure to you.

First I'd like to acknowledge the experts who reviewed my manuscript and/or shared their knowledge.

- Dr. Christine Snow, former Director of the Bone Research Laboratory at Oregon State University
- Dr. Mary Jane Gray, ACOG, Pioneer of Women's Health, Professor Emeritus
- Dr. Ken Sansome, Family Medicine Practitioner
- Dr. Frank Heresco, Diplomat of the American Board of Chiropractic Orthopedics
- Dr. Elizabeth Waldron, Geriatrician
- Dr. Christopher J. Bayne, Comparative Immunologist

Special thanks also to my editors. Your guidance and suggestions have made this book clear and concise and I trust the readers will appreciate your help as much as I did.

- Ruth B. Arendt, MA, MSW, author of <u>Stress and Your Child</u>, <u>Trust Building With Children Who Hurt</u>, and <u>Helping Children Grieve</u>
- Connie Sansome, Ph.D, author of <u>Minnesota Underfoot</u>, <u>Quarrywood Journal</u>, and <u>Minnesota in Maps: A Trailblazer Atlas</u>
- LaRea Dennis Johnston, Ph.D, author of <u>Aquatic and Wetland Plants of Oregon With Vegetative Key</u> and <u>Commonly Cultivated and Native Oregon Plants Toxic To Domesticated Animals</u>
- Cindy Hereford, copyeditor extraordinaire
- Berkeley Bayne, international traveler
- My writer's group: C. Lill Ahrens, editor, author, artist; Ange Crawford, author; Kathy Dixon, author; Ellen Beier, illustrator and author

And finally, special thanks to my graphics design mentors. I couldn't have done this without your help.

- Betty Orwick and Jessica Hodgson

Forward
by Dr. Frank Heresco

With the benefits of new technologies, new medications, alternative/complementary health care, and better knowledge of lifestyle activities, we are living much longer than our grandparents did. In the year 1900, the average lifespan for Americans was 49 years. The current expected length of life is 77.6 years and there are about 70,500 Americans over the age of 100. According to the University of Texas, by the year 2050, 800,000 Americans will be over 100 years old. It should be noted that as we live longer, diseases generally reserved for the elderly are on the rise. Skeletal function issues are currently the most significant reason for impairment of the elderly population. Spinal compression fractures, hip fractures, arthritis in the joints, and debilitating back pain are now commonplace. The timing of this book is impeccable. If you plan on living into your 80s, 90s, or past 100 years old, it is imperative that you take action now to improve your musculoskeletal health so you can enjoy a long and active life.

Living the BONES Lifestyle is an outstanding guide for proper bone health. The author, Cindy Killip, has done a wonderful job of taking a very complicated and often confusing subject and presenting it in a simple and feasible format. The advice given in this entertaining and informative book is gently motivating, understandable, and practical. As a health care provider, I would also mention that it is accurate. By following this recipe for good bone health you can avoid some of the most devastating pain and disability issues imaginable.

This book and its contents are near and dear to me. As a practicing chiropractor for over thirty years, I have had a front row seat witnessing how miserable osteoporosis can be. I want all of my patients to know this material: men 60 years and older, women 40 years and older, mothers who can teach these bone lifestyle choices to their children. Don't wait until you have advanced osteoporosis to begin practicing these simple lifestyle activities. Although they will still help at the advanced stage, you will be fighting the proverbial uphill battle. It is best to start a decade or more before bone loss. Osteoporosis is an insidious condition, but preventative medicine is smart medicine.

This is a must read for all of us. I promise you will be glad you did.

Frank Heresco, DC, DABCO

This Book Is For YOU!

Are you concerned about osteoporosis or osteopenia? Do you know which exercises and foods are best for your bones and why? Are you giving your bones all the attention they deserve?

This book, *Living The* BONES *Lifestyle: A Practical Guide To Conquering The Fear Of Osteoporosis*, will teach you the basics of bone health. It describes the structure, function, and life cycle of your bones and explains what it means to have low bone mineral density. Most importantly, it offers solutions to prevent or manage osteoporosis. Bones are living, dynamic organs that require lifelong attention. This book will teach you how to take care of your bones so you can enjoy them throughout your life.

By now you have probably heard that a calcium-rich diet is important for strong bones and know that there are medications available to treat osteoporosis. Marketing dollars have helped get this message out loud and clear through the media and the medical community. To their credit, the pharmaceutical and insurance companies have brought awareness to a serious problem – more than 40 million Americans have low bone mass and a quarter of them have osteoporosis. In fact it has been estimated that osteoporosis is associated with at least 1.5 million fractures per year. This awareness has led to improved research and screening, as well as medications and supplements that can help slow bone loss.

Unfortunately the message that consumers get is too often fear-driven. We are told that "osteoporosis is a disease that causes bones to become porous, gradually making them weaker and more brittle. Low bone mineral density may lead to fractures as this 'silent disease' progresses and, if you fracture a vertebra or hip, you may face long hospital stays, immobility, and a loss of independence." Just hearing that message leads to a feeling of vulnerability, so it's no surprise that when a person is told that she/he has "brittle bones," fear sets in, and with it a desire to prevent fractures at all costs.

Around the world, scientists have been studying the skeletal system and diseases that affect it to try to gain a clearer understanding of what actually goes on in the skeleton. Their research shows that a balanced lifestyle that includes exercise, vitamin supplements, and a variety of nutritious foods builds strong bones – even if you already have osteoporosis. Unfortunately this part of the message isn't getting relayed. In fact, when diagnosed with low bone mineral density, most people feel fragile and fear breaking a bone with a wrong movement or fall. Instead of proactively adding safe bone-building exercises, their fear encourages them to decrease activity levels and move cautiously.

Part of the reason the whole message isn't getting out is that the results of scientific studies can be confusing and conflicting. Researchers are trying to understand the why's, how's, and what if's of bone health, but the information is overwhelming, often published in obscure journals, and sometimes contradictory. Some of this confusion is due to the complexity of the skeletal system. There is much to consider, and scientists can only focus on one area at a time. Each study's results can explain only a small piece of the puzzle.

In the study of osteoporosis alone, there are hundreds of questions that must be answered, including: Why do some people develop osteoporosis and others don't? What are the causes of osteoporosis? Why do bones fracture? How can we prevent fractures, or if they occur, how can we best treat them? How does bone break down and rebuild itself? How can we facilitate bone remodeling? Is there a way to prevent osteoporosis?

Furthermore, we are trying to understand how lifestyles affect bone strength. Some of this research includes the effects of vitamins and minerals on bone mineralization and how exercise correlates to the function of specialized bone cells. Researchers want to understand exactly how food choices and different types of exercise affect the skeletal system. These studies sub-divide the research even further.

Obviously this book will not be able to cover everything that has been learned about bones. My goal in writing this book is to "put the meat on the bones" so to speak. I want to give you the gift of knowledge and make the material easy to understand and accessible to everyone. I have spent years studying this subject, analyzing and reviewing the research, and helping people put it to use in their daily routines. For more than a decade, I have taught workshops and fitness classes, and trained one-on-one with clients who are dealing with osteopenia or osteoporosis.

I am interested in how lifestyle affects bone health. As we live longer, how can we maintain strong bones? What lifestyle choices help prevent and manage osteoporosis? Can we build denser bones? If so, would that be enough or do we need to build stronger bones? And based on the available research, how can we best do that? I don't intend to diagnose or treat osteoporosis with this book. Instead, it is offered as an educational resource for you – to help you understand how your bones function, to help you evaluate your situation, and to guide you on the path to a bone-healthy lifestyle.

I decided to write this book because I see a hunger for information on this subject. In 1999, I started teaching a fitness class I call Building

Bones and Balance©. It is based on research that proved certain exercises have a positive effect on bone mineral density. During class, I often get questions related to bone mineral density tests, nutrition, supplements, and medication. It became obvious that osteoporosis is a confusing subject for many people; so in order to answer their questions, I began extensive research in these areas as well. Through the years, the most common questions I have been asked about the program are, "Is there a book that tells me everything you are teaching?" and, "Can you please write this down for me so I can share it with my sister (mom, brother, etc)?" So that is what I have done.

I have narrowed the wealth of information down to five simple steps that can help you build strong bones, what I call the BONES Lifestyle©. This book will provide you with practical solutions for developing healthy bones no matter how old you are; and healthy bones are strong bones. There is no one-size-fits-all-buy-a-fish-and-eat-today solution to bone health but there are simple steps you can take. My goal is to teach you how to fish with knowledge so you can stand up straight and keep fishing throughout your lifetime.

This book is for those of you who have asked for it and have been waiting patiently. It is for anyone who wants to preserve their bones and improve their quality of life. I firmly believe that a balanced lifestyle is the key to lifelong health and it's never too late to bring your life into balance. It makes no difference how old you are or what your fitness level: if you are interested in preventing or managing osteoporosis, you can benefit from The BONES Lifestyle©.

DISCLAIMER

The information provided in this book is intended solely for educational purposes and should not be relied upon for diagnosis, treatment, or care. Before you begin any exercise program or change your diet, supplements, or medications, discuss your situation with your physician and/or licensed health-care practitioner and make sure you understand your limitations, risk factors, and test results.

Correct technique and body position are important when performing the exercises described in this book. Therefore, it is recommended that you consult with a physical therapist or personal trainer to evaluate your technique. If a movement hurts, don't do it.

The author, publisher, and all of the references cited shall be free from responsibility should any injuries occur as a result of following these recommendations, performing these exercises, or taking medication or supplements.

The Bare Bones

If I asked why you have bones, what would your answer be? Most people hear that question and picture a skeleton providing internal structure for the body. If that was your response, you are correct — your bones are the primary structural support for your body. They protect delicate organs including your heart, lungs, and brain. They work closely with your nerves and muscles to help you sit, stand, and move. In fact, your bones are so important as a support structure that if even one of them is damaged, your posture, mobility, or in some cases, even your life could be jeopardized.

What many people don't know is that bones are also living, dynamic organs that operate as a manufacturing and storage facility. A steady supply of nutrients into and out of your bones enables your body to produce almost two–and–a–half million red blood cells per second in your bone marrow, which is located in open spaces inside the center of the bones. The bone tissue itself stores numerous minerals, including calcium, phosphorus, and magnesium set within a matrix made mostly of protein collagen. These minerals are tiny crystals that are building blocks for the bones, but they are also used by the rest of the body for other essential functions. The minerals are constantly flowing from the bone tissue to the bloodstream and back into the bone tissue through a series of blood vessels.

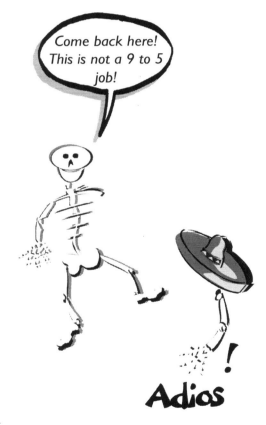

Your bones work a 24–hour shift, seven days a week. Hopefully they never decide to take a vacation.

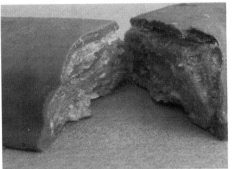

Bones make up less than 20% of your body weight while muscles make up almost 50%.

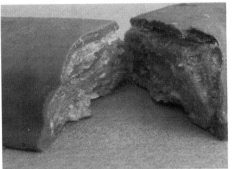

A bone looks like a Butterfinger® candy bar.

One cubic inch of healthy cortical bone can support between 18,000 and 24,000 pounds. That's equivalent to 50 pianos!

Picture Your Bone as a Candy Bar

An adult body has 206 bones that all totalled weigh only about 20 pounds. They maintain this sturdy yet lightweight structure with a unique design comprised of two types of bone tissue — **cortical** and **trabecular**. Both types of bone tissue play a role in support, manufacturing and storage, but they look different. Cortical bone tissue is a smooth shell, usually found on the outside of bone. Trabecular bone tissue is a sponge–like inner structure of bone. To put it simply, most bones look like a Butterfinger® candy bar. If you've ever enjoyed a Butterfinger, you know they have a smooth, dense chocolate coating encasing a "crispety, crunchety, peanut–buttery" inside that is more porous.

The smooth "chocolatey" shell of cortical bone is dense and compact — no more than 8 millimeters at its thickest. This type of bone tissue accounts for about 75% of your total bone mineral density. Under magnification, the cross–section of cortical bone has tiny, circular canals that look like fingerprints in the chocolate. These fingerprints, called **osteons**, are actually spherical layers of bone tissue packed tightly together. In the center of each osteon is a tiny hole that allows blood vessels to carry minerals to and from the

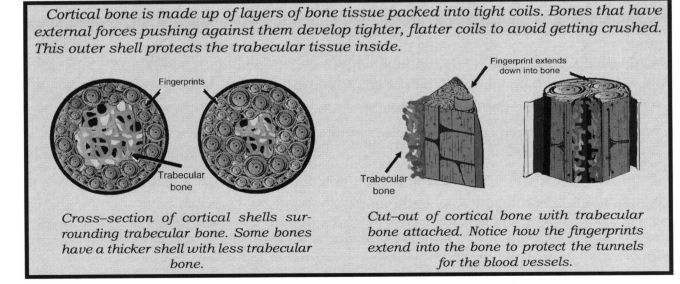

Cortical bone is made up of layers of bone tissue packed into tight coils. Bones that have external forces pushing against them develop tighter, flatter coils to avoid getting crushed. This outer shell protects the trabecular tissue inside.

Fingerprints

Trabecular bone

Fingerprint extends down into bone

Trabecular bone

Cross–section of cortical shells surrounding trabecular bone. Some bones have a thicker shell with less trabecular bone.

Cut–out of cortical bone with trabecular bone attached. Notice how the fingerprints extend into the bone to protect the tunnels for the blood vessels.

bone cells. The concentric structure of osteons provides strength. A strong cement–like outer wall around each osteon makes it difficult for cracks to spread.

Protected inside the cortical shell is the trabecular bone tissue which stores the remaining 25% of your bone's minerals. It is spongy, porous and lightweight. At a distance, trabecular bone resembles the porous crispy center of a Butterfinger candy bar. But under magnification, you see a honeycomb structure that looks more like a beehive, with pieces of open latticework that are thinner than a pencil lead. Arranged in rows along the lines of the greatest mechanical stress, they have the ability to transfer a load across the bone. This keeps the bones light in weight yet remarkably strong. Without one of the lattices, the whole structure will be weaker but can still bear the load placed on the bone.

The Design of Strength

Both types of bone are necessary for strength and function. Cortical bone tissue is stronger than trabecular bone tissue, so it provides a great deal of your bones' strength, but the geometric structure of trabecular bone is essential for support and functionality. A loss of just one tenth of core trabecular bone substantially weakens the whole bone and affects its ability to withstand impact.

In 1866 a Swiss engineer named Karl Cullman saw the head of a femur bone that had been cut in half lengthwise. "Why, that's my crane!" he exclaimed. The pattern of latticework in the trabecular bone looked just like the pattern of girders in a heavy duty crane he had recently designed for a loading dock. Cullman observed the connection between nature and structural design. Like nature, he had built along the lines of stress.

Taking their cues from nature, engineers understand the value of geometric support. Hexagons, like those found in a honeycomb, are a common support system found in nature, engineering, art,

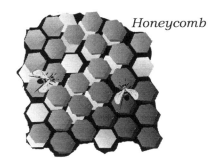
Honeycomb

Trabecular bone
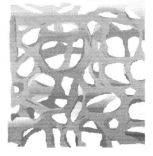

Under magnification, trabecular bone looks like a honeycomb.

> *The trabecular bone of the hip can withstand forces up to six times your body's weight.*

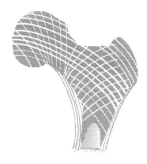

Trabecular tissue in the head of a femur bone grows in a pattern that provides the greatest strength to resist the stresses placed on that bone.

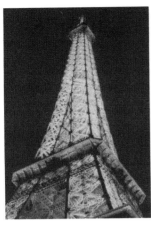

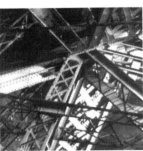

Engineering mimics nature. The crisscrossing struts of the Eiffel Tower resemble the latticework of trabecular bone.

Eiffel Tower photographs © Kathy Dixon

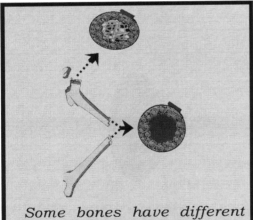

Some bones have different structures in different parts of the bone. For example, in the femur bone, the round head and neck have trabecular bone encased within the outer shell of cortical bone but the center shaft of the bone is just a hollow tube of cortical bone with no trabecular bone inside.

and architecture. Triangular trusses, often used in bridges and buildings, feature straight struts interconnected into triangular units, providing versatility and stability to the design. A famous example of building with geometric struts is the Eiffel Tower, completed in 1889. The crisscrossing struts in the tower resemble the latticework of trabecular bone.

All bones have an outer shell made of cortical tissue, but the proportions of cortical to trabecular tissue vary from one bone to the next, depending on the bone's function. In some cases the "chocolatey" cortical coating of a bone is thin ($\frac{1}{3}$ to $\frac{1}{2}$ millimeter), while in other bones it's thicker (up to 8 millimeters), resembling a solid chocolate bar.

Long bones, such as the femur bone of your thigh, the tibia in your lower leg, and the humerus bone in your upper arm have a tube shape with a hollow channel in the center. This tubular shape is composed of mostly dense cortical tissue. Trabecular tissue forms the ends where the bone articulates with other bones and must support off–center loads. The hollow tube shape provides exceptional strength while the open trusses of trabecular bone offer support along the lines of stress to spread compression and tension forces that occur with movement.

In general, your arm and leg bones have this shape with a greater percentage of dense cortical bone for load–bearing strength, while your spine, ribs, and the small bones in your wrists have more of the spongy trabecular tissue throughout — providing a lighter structure with strength where needed. Your pelvis contains a fairly even distribution of the two bone types.

From the visible bone that you can see and touch, to the cells, minerals, and nutrients that make up the bone tissue, bones have evolved for maximum strength and function. As a key storage facility, your bones' composition includes about two–thirds stored minerals like calcium and phosphorus (calcium phosphate). These minerals are tiny crystal building blocks that give

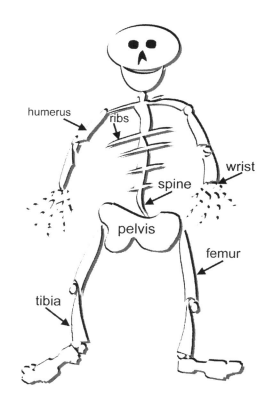

the bones their strength. The remaining third is made up of living cells and nutrients, including protein, which give the bone some elasticity so it can handle mechanical stress without shattering. The protein is actually a collagen fiber that forms a mesh–like matrix similar to the collagen in your fingernails. It serves as the foundation that holds your bones together.

The exact composition differs with each bone and with each person. It also fluctuates in each person, changing with your lifestyle and age. In 1892, German anatomist and surgeon, Julius Wolff, observed that bones in healthy people and animals adapt to the loads placed on them. Wolff's Law states that when a bone is placed under stress, it will get stronger, adapting over time to resist that type of stress. Furthermore, if the loads placed on a bone decrease, it will become weaker.

Your bones' response to forces will vary according to the direction of stress they must bear. Most bones develop strength in the direction of normal loading. In other words, if a bone must carry your body's weight, as your femur (thigh bone) must, it will be stronger in the direction of compressive forces pushing down on it. The tube–like structure of the femur allows it to carry significant loads while the direction of trabecular tresses in the neck and head of the femur are stronger along the angles of stress.

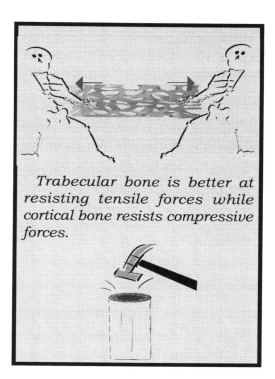

Trabecular bone is better at resisting tensile forces while cortical bone resists compressive forces.

Bendable Bones

*Scientists have found that bones can withstand at least two types of force — **compressive force** and **tensile force**. Tensile forces stretch the bone, trying to pull it apart like a game of tug-of-war. If you pull a bone from both ends, you place tension on the bone. Compressive forces come from the ends or sides of the bone and push inward toward the center of the bone. When you step on top of a soda can to crush it, you are applying compressive force. Bones must be strong enough to resist being crushed by compressive forces and flexible enough to keep from snapping under tensile forces. This is called bending strength.*

***Bending strength** is a combination of tensile strength and compressive strength. When a bone is bent, the inside of the curve is loaded under compression while the outside is loaded in tension. The side under tension is most often the first point of failure because bone is often weaker under tension than under compression. If you hold a stack of dry spaghetti noodles on either end and bend the noodles slowly, you will see this bending weakness in action. The first noodles to break are the ones to the outside of the bending angle.*

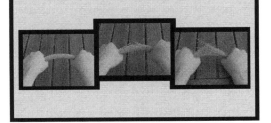

Some layers of bones have a higher percentage of collagen fibers aligned in the direction of stress to resist tension. Other layers have more mineral crystals and collagen fibers aligned across the bone to resist compressive forces. If certain bones in your body are exposed to greater compressive forces, such as the thigh bones of a gymnast who must land after a dismount, these bones will adapt to the demand and lay down a greater layer of calcium phosphate to provide strength.

Calcium in–Calcium out

The most abundant mineral in bone, calcium, is also the most well–known. Much of the research on osteoporosis and bone health focuses on calcium because calcium is also essential for normal heart and brain function, maintenance of normal blood pressure, metabolism, muscle contraction, nerve impulse transmission, and blood clotting. Every movement you make requires calcium, as does every heartbeat. It helps you maintain a strong immune system, keeps your brain sharp, reduces fatigue and even affects your eyesight! To put it simply, calcium is fundamental to life.

About 99% of your body's calcium is stored in your bone. Calcium is an essential component of bone strength. Amazingly, your body uses the remaining 1% to perform all the other necessary functions. Most of that remaining 1% flows throughout your bloodstream, keeping it available for use by the heart, muscles, nerves, and other organs.

An elaborate banking system for dietary calcium and stored calcium keeps the 1% of mobile calcium available at all times. Ideally your blood will maintain a balance between the amount of calcium you take into your body through food and supplements and the amount you lose through metabolism, sweat, urine and feces, as well as shed skin, nails, and hair. But if your blood needs additional calcium, the bank will remove it from the "mineral savings account" in your bones.

Problems arise when the balance of minerals in your bones is depleted for essential bodily

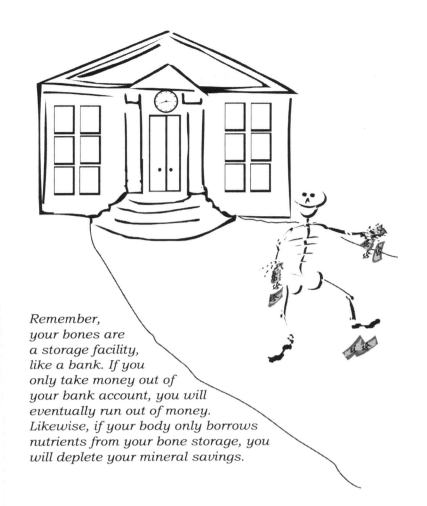

Remember,
your bones are
a storage facility,
like a bank. If you
only take money out of
your bank account, you will
eventually run out of money.
Likewise, if your body only borrows
nutrients from your bone storage, you
will deplete your mineral savings.

All together, the bones in your body contain about three pounds of calcium.

If you live with a negative calcium balance for 25 years, you will lose about $1/3$ of your peak bone density.

About 700mg of calcium flows into and out of your bones every day. That's more calcium than you'll find in two 8–ounce glasses of milk.

functions but is not replaced. You can keep the calcium bank from tapping your savings by absorbing as much of this valuable mineral as possible from your diet. This is also true for the other essential minerals that are stored in bone, specifically phosphorus, magnesium, and sodium.

Bone Masons at Work: How Does Your Bone Grow?

Your bones, like your fingernails and hair, go through a continuous cycle of growth with new cells replacing mature ones. They grow throughout your lifetime, but the rate of growth tends to be more rapid in children and slows down with age.

Bones are made of living, growing tissue that is constantly changing, but they always provide the three functions of support, manufacturing, and storage.

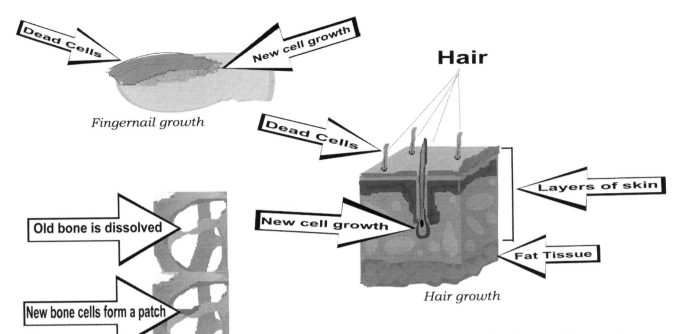

Fingernail growth

Hair

Dead Cells

New cell growth

Layers of skin

Fat Tissue

Hair growth

Old bone is dissolved

New bone cells form a patch

Bone growth

> *Your bones, hair, and fingernails all grow throughout your lifetime. But while dead tissue remains intact in fingernails and hair, in bones the dead tissue is broken down and recycled.*

As new cells grow at the base of your fingernails and hair, the older, dead cells are pushed out, forming the structures we see. Fortunately, old bone isn't pushed out quite like this. If it was, you'd be clipping your toenails and at the same time filing your femur! While dead tissue remains intact in fingernails and hair, in bone, it is broken down and the minerals are released into the blood stream. New bone tissue then replaces the dead tissue that has been released.

Basically, bone grows in much the same way that a brick wall is repaired. This bone wall is made from bricks containing minerals such as calcium and phosphorus and a mortar of living cells in a soft, fibrous protein matrix called **collagen**. Demolition experts called **osteoclasts** are at the site searching for old, cracked, or weak bricks so they can remove them from the wall. The osteoclasts form a seal on the bone's surface then "crush" the bricks by releasing an acid–like substance to break up and dissolve the "collagen mortar" in the old bone.

This demolition process creates a cavity in the bone. As the old bone breaks down, necessary nutrients, including calcium, phosphorus, and magnesium, are released into the bloodstream.

Once they've completed their job of crushing and removing old bone, the osteoclasts leave the scene by dissolving themselves.

At the same time the osteoclasts are breaking down old bone, building masons called **osteoblasts** are at work rebuilding it. The osteoblast cells come in behind the osteoclasts and fill in the cavities. They build new bone by producing a new soft collagen matrix in the cavity, then absorbing nutrients and minerals from the blood to fill it. Minerals like calcium and phosphorus provide most of the bone's strength. As the new bone forms, it responds to the stresses that are being placed on the bone and aligns the collagen fibers in the direction of stress. For bones or sections of bones that must endure significant tension, the new fibers line up with the length of the bone. For bones or sections of bones that experience more compression, the fibers line up across the bone. Once their work is done, osteoblasts change in one of the following ways:

1. They may flatten out and line up along the bone's surface as **lining cells**.

2. They may move deeper into the collagen matrix and become **osteocytes**, developing long branches that connect them to other osteocytes and lining cells.

3. They may dissolve like the osteoclasts.

If they evolve into either lining cells or osteocytes, they become part of the new bone and help direct bone remodeling. The primary job of osteocytes appears to be to sense mechanical strain and that of lining cells appears to be to release calcium from bone if more is needed in the blood.

The process of breakdown and growth, called **remodeling**, is dynamic and takes place on the surface of each bone, whether its tissue is cortical or trabecular. We do not completely understand the process of remodeling, but we do know it is an important system that protects bone strength. It appears that bone cells are added to areas of the bones that are under stress and removed from areas that aren't. How this occurs is not totally

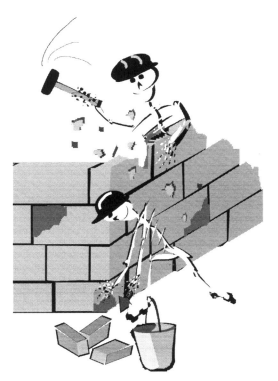

Demolition experts busily break down old bone while bone masons are at work building new bone.

There can actually be up to 10 million sites of bone breaking down and building up in your body at any given moment, and it is estimated that about 10% of your entire skeleton is replaced each year.

> *One study done on pigs showed that the bones of an adult pig contained none of the calcium that was present when it was a piglet, indicating that the adult pigs' skeletons had completely regenerated at least once during their lifetime.*

clear. Some studies suggest that a form of electrical stimulation transfers signals from bone to bone cells. When an external electrical current is applied to bone, new bone forms to a greater extent than when no current is applied. So a bone that is experiencing greater strains may request additional help by way of electrical impulses, possibly through the nervous system. This suggestion makes sense considering the close working relationship between nerves, muscles, and bones, but more research is needed in this area.

A Balanced Body

Nerves, muscles, and bones are only part of a balanced body. A balanced body is a healthy body with all systems functioning at their best. Your nails, hair, and bones are each specialized, complex systems that are carefully choreographed to function throughout life. Working in concert with all the other systems in your body, such as digestion and circulation, they remain strong and healthy as long as your body remains in balance.

When your body is in balance, your smallest toenail and finest hair will receive the nutrients necessary to be strong and healthy. Unfortunately, necessary functions in the body sometimes slip out of balance, and the effects can be seen in your nails, hair, and bones. A decrease in your bone strength, a change in your hair's texture or an about–face in your finger or toenail shape or appearance can indicate a vitamin or mineral deficiency or other imbalance within your body.

OsteoWHAT?

Osteoclasts, Osteoblasts, Osteoporosis, Osteoyadda-yadda-yadda. How can you remember what all these words mean? Well, for starters, 'osteon' is the Greek word for bone and 'osteo' is the Greek prefix meaning to do with bone. So we know that all these words have something to do with bones.

- **Osteon** is the principle organizing feature of cortical bone, which is the compact outer shell of bone. An osteon is actually circular layers of bone tissue packed tightly together. In the center of each osteon is a tiny hole that allows blood vessels to carry nutrients and oxygen to and from the bone cells.
- **'Clast'** is the Greek root meaning to break or break into pieces. An easy way to remember this is to think of the 'c' in clast standing for crush. **Osteoclasts** are living bone cells that crush old bone and release nutrients into the blood. They do this by creating a seal on the surface of bone and secreting acids and enzymes that dissolve the bone. As the bone dissolves, nutrients and minerals are released into the bloodstream. When their work is done, the osteoclasts die off by dissolving themselves.
- **'Blast'** is the Greek root meaning formative cell or layer or bud, as in a flower bud. Think of the 'b' in blast standing for build. **Osteoblasts** are living cells that absorb nutrients from the blood and build new bone. As osteoblasts mature, they become part of the new bone as either **osteocytes** or **lining cells**, or they die off like the osteoclasts. If they become lining cells, they flatten into pancake–shaped cells and line the outer surface of the bone. They are responsible for releasing calcium from the bone if the blood suddenly needs more and they help with the initiation of bone remodeling. Lining cells communicate with osteocytes. Osteocytes are mature osteoblasts that are surrounded by collagen matrix. Located deep within the bone tissue, these cells have branches that allow them to contact other bone cells and sense any mechanical strain on the bone. Although their exact role is not yet known, it is thought that they direct bone remodeling and the repair of damaged bone.
- **'Porosis'** is a Latin suffix that means porous. So **osteoporosis** literally means porous bones. If your body doesn't make enough bone or you lose too much bone, you may develop osteoporosis. The bone–building cycle shifts out of balance and the osteoclasts crush more bone than the osteoblasts can build. It causes weaker bones that can lead to bone fractures.
- **'Penia'** is a Greek suffix meaning poverty or lack of. **Osteopenia** means lower than normal bone mineral density. It is the first stage of bone loss and a warning that osteoporosis may be on the horizon.

2

The Opponent: Osteoporosis

An unfortunate fact of life is that, as you age, your bones weaken. This weakness comes from multiple factors, and results in porous and brittle bones.

Bone mineral density naturally starts its decrease during middle age. The loss of bone mineral density makes bones more porous. Problems may occur if your bone mineral density decreases at a younger age, at a faster rate than normal, or never fully increased to a maximum peak bone density.

At the same time your bones are losing density, the balance between the mineral crystals and the protein collagen fiber matrix is also changing. Bones increase their percentage of mineral content with age and decrease their percentage of collagen. It is this imbalance of collagen to mineral that contributes to the brittleness of bones.

A strong bone must have balanced growth with enough mineral content for hardness and enough collagen for flexibility. If your bones were made of only mineral crystals, they would be very hard, but brittle, and they would fracture easily. If they were made of only protein collagen fiber matrix, your bones would be very flexible, and would stretch, bend and bounce like rubber, but they wouldn't support your body.

With osteoporosis, this collagen-mineral balance is upset by an impairment of the bone remodeling process. The feedback system does not

> *Bones must be able to resist tensile, compressive and bending forces. They do so with a combination of mineral crystals, collagen fibers and a jelly–like matrix of protein and sugars.*
>
> *The composition of bone is similar to that of fiberglass. Both are classified as composite materials, meaning they are made up of two or more simpler materials. Fiberglass consists of fine fibers of glass embedded in a jelly–like plastic resin. The glass provides strength to resist tensile forces and the resin provides flexibility to resist compressive forces. Combined, they make fiberglass an excellent building material that can resist forces that stretch it, bend it and compress it. Although bone is weaker than fiberglass, it serves its purpose well — to provide support and protection for the body.*

> *The most common way any bone, healthy or osteoporotic, breaks, is by bending. As bones become more brittle with age or osteoporosis, they lose much of their ability to resist bending. To make matters worse, because of the uneven weakening of bone structure, an osteoporotic bone is also more likely to break when subjected to compressive forces. This can be seen when an osteoporotic vertebra collapses.*

function correctly, so bones erode but don't rebuild with balanced protein collagen and mineral content.

Remember, there is a continuous flow of minerals both into and out of the bone. To release minerals into the blood stream, the protein collagen matrix is dissolved. Normally, new protein collagen and mineral are added to replace that which is dissolved and released. But if new bone tissue isn't formed at the same rate that old bone tissue is dissolved, the bone mineral content decreases and the bone may become porous. If the new bone is formed with too much mineral content and doesn't contain enough protein collagen to balance the minerals, it may become brittle — hard but not flexible. Either way, the bone will break more easily with less impact.

Studies to determine the brittleness of femur bones measured the amount of energy required to break the bone. Strips of bone were cut from the femurs of patients of various ages who had died from causes unrelated to bone strength. It was found that the mineral content of the bone samples actually increased with age, and the bones with higher calcium content contained less protein collagen and were more brittle. Bone from elderly people required one-third the amount of energy to break as did samples of the same size from children. In other words, elderly bone is three times as brittle as young bone but has a higher mineral content. This suggests that it is lower protein collagen content in relation to higher mineral content that contributes to the brittleness of older bones.

Modeling

During childhood, the osteoblasts (building masons) work faster than the osteoclasts (bone crushers), and new bone is formed at a faster rate than old bone is destroyed. During this period, bones change shape and grow bigger and stronger. This process of growth is called **bone modeling**. Sometime during your 20's or 30's, you hit your peak bone mineral density. This peak density and the age it is reached will vary from person to person. A number of factors determine your peak bone mineral density. Some of these factors include gender, body size, genetics, diet, medications, your age at puberty, and the amount of weight–bearing activity you did during your bone–growth years.

Also contributing to the variations in bone mineral density is that each person's bone structure is unique. The trabeculae (lattice crosspieces) in trabecular bone vary in size, number, separation, and shape from person to person. Not only will this affect bone density measurements, but this can also have a major impact on bone strength and functionality. Bone density is not equal to bone strength. As we saw earlier, the arrangement of trabeculae plays a major role in bone strength. The same applies to cortical bone. In some cases, the cortical shell will be thinner indicating lower overall bone density, but the cells will be arranged

Bone Strength

Although you may see the phrases "bone mass," "bone density," and "bone strength" used interchangeably, they do not mean the same thing.

- ***Bone mass*** *refers to how much bone there is in an object. Your bone mass is the amount of bone you have in your body.*
- ***Bone density***, *on the other hand, refers to the amount of bone tissue per cubic centimeter of bones (measured as g/cm^3). This can be confusing. A good way to visualize this is to picture brown sugar in a measuring cup. If the brown sugar is loosely scooped into the cup, the density will be small and less brown sugar will fit into the space than if it is compacted into the same container. Compacted, the same amount of brown sugar (mass) will occupy less volume and consequently carry a greater density. This is because when it is not compacted, the brown sugar contains a lot of air space between the individual granules.*
- ***Bone mineral density (BMD)*** *is an estimate of actual bone density. It is difficult to determine actual bone density so instead we measure bone mineral density, which is the amount of minerals, such as calcium, in a square centimeter of bone. This is measured as g/cm^2.*
- ***Bone strength*** *refers to the power of the bone to resist force or strain. It is the resistance to fracture. Bone strength is dependent on sufficient bone density, an adequate balance of minerals for hardness, and protein collagen for flexibility. A strong bone will resist both compressive and tensile forces. The goal of the "BONES Lifestyle" program is to develop strong bones that won't fracture when subjected to normal forces or strain.*

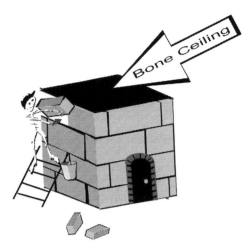

Bone modeling is the growth that occurs during childhood and young adulthood. New bone is added during this phase.

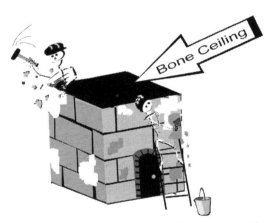

Bone remodeling is the regrowth that occurs in adulthood. No new bone is added but old bone is replaced during this phase.

in such a way as to provide greater strength than a thicker shell.

Once your bone mineral density has peaked, you have reached your "bone ceiling", and the process of bone growth changes. Modeling ends and remodeling begins as the osteoclasts (bone crushers) break down the old bone and osteoblasts (building masons) build new bone at a relatively equal rate. Additional bone is no longer added, but old, weak, and damaged bone is replaced by new bone. You can replace bone that is lost but you cannot increase your bone mineral density beyond your ceiling.

When Construction Goes Wrong

In some cases the remodeling cycle remains equal as we age, osteoclasts and osteoblasts balance each other out so there is no net loss of bone. But more often the remodeling cycle changes with age and the mineral density of the bones gradually decreases. This decline is normal although the speed at which it occurs varies from person to person. Middle–aged women typically lose between zero and three percent of their bone mineral content per year. The loss tends to stay below one percent for middle–aged men.

There are three main imbalances that lead to bone loss.

1. The entire remodeling rate may increase and throw things out of balance.
2. Osteoclast activity (bone crushing) may increase and the osteoblasts (bone builders) can't keep up.
3. Osteoblast activity (bone building) may slow down or stop completely so that as mature cells die new ones don't replace them.

When the remodeling cycle is out of balance in the dense outer shell of cortical bone (remember the chocolate part of a Butterfinger candy bar?), the tissue becomes more porous and less dense, decreasing the bone's strength. When it is out of balance in the trabecular tissue (the "crispety, crunchety, peanut buttery" inside of the candy bar that resembles the structural support of the Eiffel Tower), the thickness and connectivity of the struts that make up the triangular trusses are affected.

Remember, this ongoing process of breakdown and buildup always takes place in the tissue that is located on the outer surface of bone because osteoclasts form a seal on the bone's surface then release their dissolving acids and enzymes. Since the lattice shape of trabecular tissue has more surface area than the flat shape of cortical tissue, there is more bone available to break down in this type of tissue. Therefore, bones with a higher percentage of trabecular, or spongy, tissue are the ones that are affected first and most. In fact, you lose trabecular bone twice as fast as cortical bone. If this mineral and protein collagen loss is not built back up at a similar rate, the struts that support the trabecular bone become thinner or disappear completely.

If the struts begin to thin but the basic structure remains intact, it still has some strength but the bone is at a greater risk of fracturing. This is considered osteopenia. With osteopenia, 10% to 25% of peak bone density has been lost.

> *Bone remodeling takes place on the surface of bone. Trabecular bone has a greater surface area on all of its supporting struts, making up about 70% of your bones' total surface area. Therefore, it's not surprising that these bones are the first to show signs of weakening. Because of its more compact nature, cortical bone is generally not affected until later in life. When it is affected, cortical bone becomes thinner and more porous with larger cavities.*

	Cortical Bone	Trabecular Bone
% of total skeletal mass	80%	20%
% of bone that has surface area	33%	67%
Porosity	Low	High
Remodeling rate	Slow	Rapid

> *While bone is in the process of remodeling, the mineral content is low until enough minerals have been absorbed by the collagen matrix; so new bone has a lower mineral content than older bone.*

Without intervention, the imbalanced remodeling can lead to a greater loss of tissue leaving very thin trabecular struts with larger spaces between them, or even eliminating some of the struts. When this happens, there isn't enough support for normal activity. This is considered osteoporosis. If you've been diagnosed with osteoporosis, you've lost at least 25% of your peak bone density.

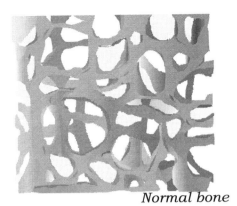

Normal bone

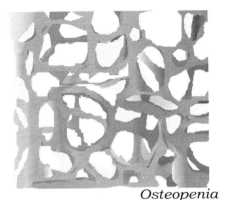

Osteopenia

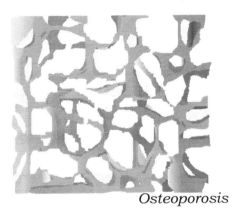

Osteoporosis

Imagine what would happen to the Eiffel Tower if some of its crisscrossing braces were removed. You wouldn't want to be sightseeing from the top platform on that day! That weakening is basically what is happening to trabecular bone that is affected by osteoporosis.

As the bone architecture breaks down throughout your body, one or more bones will have greater bone mineral deficits than the others. These are the bones that are most likely to fracture. You may have normal bone mineral density in some bones and low bone mineral density in others.

For some people, vertebral bone mineral density is low. The height and cross–section of one or more of their vertebrae may be smaller, the width of the cortical bone thinner, and/or the trabecular struts may be thinner or missing, while the hip's femoral neck shows minimal reductions in size and bone mineral density. These people tend to suffer from vertebral fractures.

People who experience hip fractures often have vertebrae of normal size with only a slight decrease in bone mineral density in the spine, but the diameter of the femoral necks in their hips may be smaller, the cortical bone in the femur may develop large cavities and the trabecular struts may become thinner or disappear. These people are at a greater risk of experiencing a hip fracture. Likewise, people who develop wrist fractures have been shown to have greater bone mineral deficits at the forearm than at the spine or hip.

Your body is unique. Each person who is affected by osteoporosis will be affected differently. It's important to understand where your greatest weaknesses are so you can take appropriate action. But keep in mind that osteoporosis is a systemic disease. It may affect one bone first, but it still affects all of the bones in your body.

Osteoporosis: It's not Just For Women

Osteoporosis affects both men and women, but for every man that is diagnosed with it, four women are diagnosed. One reason for this discrepancy is that men start off with greater bone density than women, so they have more material to work with. Men also tend to participate in more physically demanding work and play activities that require strength more than women do. Also, men in general focus less on dieting to lose weight.

While these physical and cultural influences can affect who may get osteoporosis, the main reason for the discrepancy is that unless they have a medical condition or take medication that affects bone metabolism, men don't begin to lose bone until sometime after age 60. After about age 70, both men and women lose bone density due to an age–related decrease of bone building remodeling. But while men only lose bone during these later years, women experience greater bone loss after **menopause** as well. So women experience significant bone loss during two periods of their lives — around the time of menopause, and again around age 70.

Different hormones between the sexes play a significant role. In men, **androgens**, especially **testerone**, are the main triggers for the bone remodeling cycle. In women, the triggers are **estrogen** and **progesterone**. While androgens and testosterone levels stay relatively stable throughout a man's life, declining slowly as men age, female estrogen levels decline rapidly and significantly during menopause.

Estrogen increases the remodeling rate and suppresses the activity of the osteoclasts (bone crushing cells). As estrogen levels decrease during and after menopause, the osteoclasts' performance and lifespan increase, giving them more opportunity to destroy bone. The decrease in estrogen also decreases the lifespan of the osteoblasts (bone–building cells) so less bone is created. For women, decline in bone density is greatest during this period.

During the five to ten years following menopause, bone loss occurs at a rate of about three to five percent per year. Because of its greater surface area, most of the bone that is lost during this time is trabecular bone. After the post–menopause years, the rate of bone loss typically

> *Women can lose up to 20% of their bone density after menopause.*

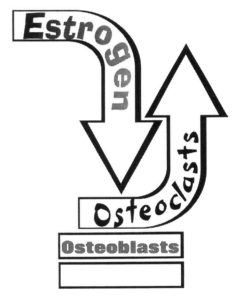

As the amount of estrogen in your body declines during menopause, the activity of the osteoclasts (bone crushers) increases while that of the osteoblasts (bone builders) remains about the same. As a result, more bone is broken down than built up.

slows down to about one percent per year until age–related bone loss increases around age 70. Women older than 70 are at a greater risk of bone mineral loss if they smoke, become less active, or are deficient in vitamin D.

Age–related bone loss in men is typically a result of less bone being formed rather than an increase in the amount of bone being broken down. Since men don't lose bone at a rapid rate during mid–life, trabeculae are usually better preserved in men's bones than in women's. Men typically begin losing bone mineral density around age 60 at a rate of only 0.2 to 0.5 percent per year. Men who are 75 or older with a slight build are the most likely to have osteoporosis. If they have lost more than 5 percent of their body weight during the previous four years, currently smoke or are physically inactive, men's risk of fracture will increase. Smoking is the main lifestyle risk factor for osteoporosis in males. Osteoporosis in younger males is often linked to another disease or medication.

The deterioration of bone mineral density can be devastating, and often strikes without warning, but there is some hopeful news. Doctors can measure your bone mineral density so you can get an idea of how dense your bones are, and whether you may be at risk for osteoporosis. Your current bone mineral density is one indicator of a faulty remodeling process although there is some debate as to whether bone mineral density is an accurate predictor of fracture.

If osteoporosis is defined as a "risk factor" for fracture as it came to be defined in the 1990's then bone mineral density is a useful measurement. But if we define osteoporosis as it was originally defined — a condition that leads to fragile bones that fracture easily — then there are many risk factors involved, and a simple measurement of your bone mineral density can not definitively diagnose it. At the time of this printing, the best tool available to measure bone mineral density is a machine called a DEXA or DXA. This is the acronym for an enhanced form of x–ray technology

> *Bone mineral density that is significantly lower than normal is called osteopenia or osteoporosis, depending on the severity. A loss of 10% to 25% of your peak bone mineral density due to an unbalanced remodeling cycle is classified as* **osteopenia**. *A loss of more than 25% of your peak bone mineral density is classified as* **osteoporosis**.

called dual–energy x–ray absorptiometry. I will discuss this in more detail in chapter 5.

According to the National Osteoporosis Foundation (NOF), in 2006 about 55% of Americans ages 50 and older were affected by low bone mineral density as compared to the normal adult population. Because osteoporosis has the potential to affect so many women, the NOF recommends bone density testing for all women over age 65 and all women under the age of 65 who have one or more additional risk factors for osteoporosis, not including menopause.

The most important of these additional risk factors are familial history of spine or hip fracture and thinness — typically women who weigh less than 125 pounds. Although there are no current guidelines for testing bone mineral density in men, they should discuss their risk factors with a doctor to determine if a bone density test is a good idea.

Now that we are living longer lives, osteoporosis as a *risk factor* for future bone fracture is affecting more people, and is becoming a more common health concern. However, osteoporosis as a *disease* that impairs the bone's remodeling cycle causing fragile bones, is much less common. Either way, the numbers are worth acknowledging because fragility fractures are a cause of both physical and financial suffering for those who must endure them.

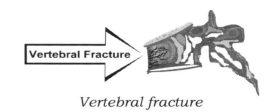

Vertebral fracture

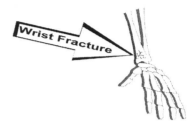

Wrist fracture

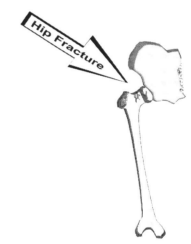

Hip fracture

Complications of Osteoporosis

Osteoporosis is called a "silent disease" because in its early stages, there are few symptoms. But during this silent decline in the mineral density and/or strength of bones, their structure is weakened. Once a bone is weakened, there is a much greater risk of fracture, often while performing daily movements as simple as getting out of bed.

Spine and Wrist Fractures

Early stages of osteoporosis affect mostly the trabecular tissue. Compression fractures of the

When osteoporosis strikes, it is often the bones in the spine, ribs and wrist that are the most vulnerable because of their high percentage of trabecular tissue. Fractures of the upper section of the thigh bone (femur), in the narrow neck of trabecular tissue between the long part of the bone and the ball that connects the femur to the pelvis socket are also common. We call this a hip fracture.

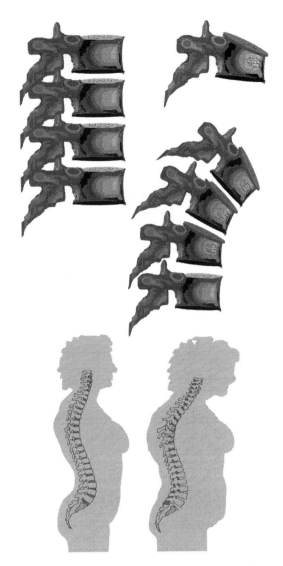

spine and fractures of the wrist are common during this period. They may occur with a minimal amount of trauma, including a cough or sneeze.

Spinal fractures are the most common type of osteoporotic fracture. They can cause significant pain, loss of mobility, poor posture, and loss of height. The spine faces considerable loads during daily life. If the vertebra is not strong enough to resist compressive forces, there is a high risk of a compressive fracture.

The most common type of vertebral fracture that occurs with osteoporosis is a wedge fracture. This is a type of compression fracture where the front part of the vertebra collapses, creating a wedge shape. These fractures rarely result from a fall but occur most often when straightening the back after rounding it forward. If more than one vertebra suffers a wedge fracture, the spine will collapse forward. This may press your chest toward the front of your hips, causing digestive problems or difficulty breathing.

Other types of compression fractures include crush fractures in which the back of the vertebra or the entire vertebra collapses and biconcave fractures which affect the central portion of the vertebra leaving the front and back edges intact. Although the number may vary between individuals, a bone density of $110mg/cm^3$ is considered the minimum density required for a vertebra to avoid fractures. The vertebrae that are most likely to experience a compressive fracture are the ones located in the upper lumbar region and mid to lower thoracic region of your spine. That's roughly the middle and lower part of your back.

Hip Fractures

In people around 70 years old, the bone loss progresses to include both trabecular and com-

If more than one vertebra suffers a wedge fracture, the spine may collapse forward causing a forward rounding of the back. The vertebra that are most likely to suffer from this type of fracture are in the middle and lower part of your spine. The term dowager's hump is often used to describe multiple fractures in the middle to upper region of the spine creating a humpback appearance.

Normal Vertebra   *Wedge Fracture*   *Crush Fracture*   *Biconcave Fracture*

pact (cortical) bone. Hip fractures are often a result of age–related changes in cortical bone so
they are more common in older individuals than
in younger people. However, they can still occur
in younger people.

Hip fractures are a major complication of osteoporosis. They can lead to a loss of mobility
and independence. At least half of the people who
sustain a hip fracture will require assistance with
daily activities, and the fatality rate within the
first year after a hip fracture is estimated to be
between 15% and 20%.

The risk of a hip fracture increases significantly as people age. Since a hip fracture can be
so devastating, researchers have looked into why
the risk increases so much with age. What they
have learned is that a fracture of the femoral neck
of the hip may have more to do with structural
changes that come with aging than simply a loss
of bone mineral density.

Aging causes a natural decrease in cortical
bone on the top part of the femoral neck while the
lower part of the femoral neck actually increases
in thickness. This is because the top section of
the femoral neck does not experience much stress
when the body is upright and walking but the
section underneath does. Years of walking and
standing in an upright position causes the bone to
adapt and creates an imbalance of bone strength.

A fall onto the hip places high stress on the
upper section of the femoral neck. Picture an alu-
minum soda can on its side, and imagine someone stepping on it. This is how the femoral neck
responds to the impact of a fall. Combined with
the fact that elderly people tend to fall more often,
this structural change is a more likely cause of
hip fractures in elderly people than a loss of bone
mineral density.

With both hip and spinal fractures, you are
likely to experience a loss of balance, a limited
range of motion and a loss of functional strength.
If one fracture occurs, you may develop a fear of
falling which ironically can lead to more falls and

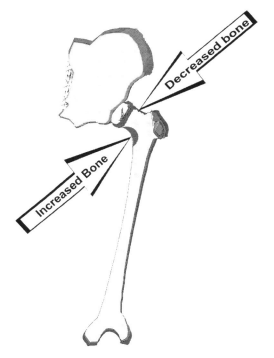

*Fractures of the femoral neck
at the hip may have more to do
with structural changes that
come with aging than simply a
loss of bone mineral density.*

more fractures. Although wrist fractures may not seem as significant, they are painful and limit your ability to perform daily tasks.

Good News

The good news is that complications from osteoporosis are preventable with some simple lifestyle changes. Osteoporosis is treatable, and in many cases, reversible. If you live a bone–healthy lifestyle, you can avoid the complications that come with osteoporosis. Educate yourself about your bones' current state of health and strive to bring your body into balance because a balanced body is more often than not a healthy body. Consume a varied diet rich in vitamins and minerals; decrease stress; and exercise regularly — performing weight–bearing exercises designed to load the skeletal system.

The rest of this book will teach you how to live the **BONES** Lifestyle to prevent or manage osteoporosis.

3

The BONES Lifestyle©

The purpose of this book and of the **BONES** Lifestyle is to simplify the overwhelming amount of information out there about bone health and osteoporosis. With all the material available, it is easy to get overwhelmed and frightened. But if you can remember the word "BONES," it will be easy to recall the steps to optimal bone health. The letters of the word BONES conveniently provide an acronym that spells out the steps and (even more conveniently) follows the order of care for your bones.

Balance training

Osteoporosis tests

Nutrition

Exercise

Supplements and Medication

This chapter will introduce you to the five steps of the **BONES** Lifestyle and the remaining chapters will delve in more deeply, explaining the why's and how's of each step.

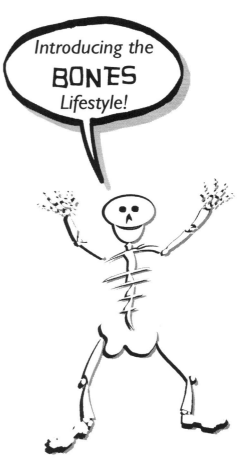

Introducing the **BONES** *Lifestyle!*

Love your bones and they will support you!

B is for Balance

Because osteoporosis weakens bone strength, and weak bones are more likely to break if you fall, the fear of falling becomes a major concern for anyone who has osteoporosis or is at risk of developing it.

Balance is affected by three senses:
- Seeing (**visual system/vision**),
- Touch (**neuromuscular system** including muscles, nerves, and the brain)
- Hearing (**vestibular system** of the inner ear).

If normal function of one of these senses is disrupted, your brain cannot clearly process the world around you, and your balance diminishes. But as long as two of the three balance senses are working correctly, your brain will override the lack of stimuli or improper messages it receives from the dysfunctional system.

For example, dizziness, which is often caused by an inner ear infection, affects balance. Your inner ear acts like a gyroscope for balance. If it has a difficult time stabilizing itself, your vestibular system will experience a sensation of movement — even if you are standing still. Your vestibular system relays this information to the brain and tells it that you are moving, but at the same time your neuromuscular system is telling your brain that you are still. This may cause you to lose your balance. However, if you focus your eyes on a point that is not moving, and stabilize your muscles, you can override this improper message from the inner ear, and stay balanced.

If you don't see clearly, you must rely on your senses of touch and hearing to create a clear picture for your brain of your body's position. If you have lost some feeling in your feet, legs, or another part of your body, you should focus more on your vision and hearing through the position of your head. You can function easily with one of the three senses out of commission, but it's much harder when two of them are down.

Unfortunately, as we age our ability to balance tends to decline. This decline is typically due to changes in the visual, neuromuscular, and vestibular systems. Other normal changes due to aging affect how your brain receives messages, and may also lead to a lack of balance. With aging you can expect a decrease in functional strength, changes in posture, less feeling in hands and feet, diminished vision or hearing, and side effects of illnesses and medications

Balance is the first step toward building stronger bones. If you are overcome by a fear of falling, you may not pursue all the avenues of good bone health. Chapter 4 will teach you how to develop better balance.

O is for Osteoporosis Tests

Because osteoporosis comes on silently and shows few symptoms, there aren't a lot of ways to know you have (or will get) this condition. The medical community has determined some key risk factors, but just because you have one or more of the risk factors doesn't mean you will develop osteoporosis. The only sure diagnosis for osteoporosis is a fracture that occurs without excessive stress or impact. Fortunately, new technology has given us techniques that can help predict whether these fractures may occur.

Tests that measure bone mineral density offer insight into your bones' state of wellness. If you learn that your bone mineral density is decreasing, you can take preventative measures and hopefully halt or reverse the trend toward weaker bones. These tests provide a strong psychological motivation to stick with your exercise and nutrition program.

As you will read in chapter 5, the best test available to measure bone mineral density at this time is the dual–energy x–ray absorptiometry (DEXA) scan. Providing a relatively accurate measurement of bone density, it is an easy, noninvasive test that delivers a very low dose of radiation and provides good results. DEXA bone scans aren't cheap — the current cost is about

$250. But if you have multiple risk factors for osteoporosis, your insurance company may pay for the test. It is a good idea to get a preliminary test to establish your baseline bone mineral density for future reference.

If your test results show low bone mineral density (BMD) and you begin treatment with medication, insurance will often cover not only a repeat scan at the end of the first year to monitor progress, but also a scan every two years after that. If cost is an issue, check with your insurance company to confirm coverage before you get the scan. If they will not pay for it, you may want to ante up and get the test anyhow. The investment into your future health and well–being will be worth it. Once you know your risk factors and potential for osteoporosis–related fractures, you can move on with the rest of your **BONES** Lifestyle.

N is for Nutrition

The medical community and media have done a good job getting the message out that a calcium–rich diet encourages strong bones. Studies show that calcium intake is essential for strong bones, and it clearly helps reduce bone loss and osteoporotic fractures in people over 65. In one study women who had an average calcium intake of 940mg/day had fewer hip fractures compared to women who had an average daily intake of 441mg. In another study, laboratory animals fed a diet that lacked sufficient calcium developed osteoporosis. Unfortunately with so much emphasis on calcium, many people don't realize that there are other nutrients that are also essential for bone health.

Simply drinking a glass of milk a day will not prevent bone fractures, although it will provide a good dose of calcium for your body's daily needs. To manage or prevent osteoporosis, you need to consume a variety of nutrients. Newer research is uncovering an assortment of vitamins and minerals that are necessary for bone strength and fracture prevention. Some of these nutrients include:

- **Calcium:** found in dairy products, soy, leafy green veggies, broccoli, fish with bones, and water.
- **Vitamin D:** absorbed through skin when exposed to sunlight; found in fatty fish, fortified milk, egg yolks, butter, and cod liver oil.
- **Magnesium:** found in nuts, legumes, whole grains, dark green veggies, seafood, and chocolate.
- **Vitamin K:** found in dark green leafy vegetables, brussels sprouts, cabbage, broccoli, and vegetable oils.
- **Zinc:** found in oysters, red meat, poultry, legumes, nuts, and whole grains.
- **Boron:** found in fruits, vegetables, nuts, and legumes.
- **Vitamin B$_{12}$:** found in red meat, poultry, fish, shellfish, eggs, milk, and fortified products.

As you can see from the list above, your bones, like the rest of your body, need a variety of foods to function at their best. In fact, at the date of this printing, at least 22 nutrients have been identified as necessary for bone health. Singling out one nutrient and eating more of that without paying attention to a balanced diet will lead to imbalances in your bones' remodeling cycle. It is best to focus on eating a variety of colorful fruits and vegetables, whole grains, fish, meat, eggs, nuts, legumes, and dairy products.

The BONES Lifestyle includes foods that are as close to their natural state as possible with skin and fiber intact. The more processed a food is, the more its nutrient content has been altered.

Processing includes cooking, mashing, and juicing as well as the more drastic practices of bleaching, stripping off the outer shell, adding chemicals, and extruding. So, for example, a whole apple is more nutritious than applesauce. Natural applesauce is more nutritious than pure apple juice.

Bone metabolism is not just a matter of nutrients in/nutrients out. It is a complex system that must balance the work of the bone crushers with that of the bone builders. There is strong evidence that diet can influence these processes, by both inhibiting the bone crushers and by encouraging the bone builders. True, calcium storage is necessary for bone density, but the process of bone remodeling is as important or more important, and this cannot be achieved without all the necessary nutrients working together. Chapter 6 discusses the nutritional aspects of bone health in more detail.

E is for Exercise

Study after study has proven that exercise is critical to healthy bones. Exercise slows bone loss and stimulates the formation of new bone tissue that is both strong and flexible, making it able to withstand the stresses of life without breaking. Many studies even suggest that it's not age that's a primary risk factor for bone loss, but it is actually a decreased level of activity that people adopt as they get older. There are typically fewer cases of osteoporosis in societies where people stay active throughout their lives.

In chapter 7 you will see that exercise can prevent, manage, and in some cases even reverse the effects of osteoporosis. Some of the most valuable studies on bone health have come from NASA–sponsored studies to determine the effects of zero gravity on astronauts' bones. The gravity–free environment causes astronauts to lose bone density, even during a short mission. This is because our bodies are designed to respond to the environment — like the chameleon who changes his colors in response to the surrounding temperature and light.

If you simulate a gravity–free environment in your lifestyle by spending too much time sitting on a chair, lying in bed, or floating in a pool, your bones will decrease in density. This is because they don't require as much strength to maintain that lifestyle. In contrast, when you exercise, the additional force of gravity pushing you downward, the impact of your feet striking the ground, or your arm swinging through a tennis stroke and striking the ball signals your bones to increase in strength so they will be able to withstand the force.

Not only do you have the forces of gravity and impact challenging your bones when you get up and move, but the contraction of your muscles also increases your bone strength. When you contract a muscle, it becomes shorter and thicker and pulls on whatever it is attached to. The muscles of your musculoskeletal system attach to tendons, which in turn, attach to bones. When you contract one of these muscles, it shortens and pulls on the bone, causing the bone to move around its joint (your elbow, for example). If you relax the muscle, it lengthens and stops pulling but it does not push the bone back into place. Muscles can only pull, so to move the bone back to its original position, an opposite muscle must contract to pull it back, thus tugging on the bone in the other direction. All this tugging keeps the remodeling system active in the same way toddlers keep their parents active!

Depending on the activities you do in your daily life, you will engage certain muscles on a regular basis. These muscles attach to the bones via tendons so they can pull on the bone to move it. Your muscles respond to exercise by getting stronger. Your bones respond to your muscles' strength by increasing in density and elasticity so they don't break when pulled by the muscle. The increase in bone strength is directly proportional to the amount of stress applied to it. If you only use some of your muscles, then only some of your bones will get stronger. If you stop exercising, you will lose the muscle strength that you gained, and you will also eventually lose much of the additional bone strength that you gained. In order to maintain the benefits of exercise, you must make it a whole-body, lifetime habit.

> *Your body adapts to the activities of your daily life. If you challenge your body with exercise, your muscles will respond by getting stronger and your bones will respond to your muscles' increased strength by increasing density and flexibility.*

> *There are about 650 muscles and 206 bones in your body. That means there about three muscles for every bone in your body. That's a lot of tugging!*

> *Muscles in your body that are contracted regularly will get stronger and contract more easily upon command. Strong muscles also tend to maintain a slightly contracted position when at rest, placing a greater load on the attached bones throughout the day.*

S is for Supplements and Medication

There is clear evidence that solid nutrition and exercise are beneficial for your bones. Combined, they can help you build strong bones, prevent osteoporosis, and even increase bone density. But what if you are doing all of that and your bone density continues to decrease, or worse, you have sustained a fragility fracture? In chapter 8 you will see that when things get way out of balance, we are fortunate to live during a time that medical science can help us live longer, healthier lives.

The S in the **BONES** Lifestyle stands for Supplements and Medication. Vitamin supplementation can help provide necessary nutrients, especially if your body doesn't absorb them well from the foods you eat or you have food sensitivities that limit your food choices. To help solve this dilemma, vitamin manufacturers are starting to make multivitamins formulated specifically for bone health.

While the nutrients in a vitamin/mineral supplement will support the bone builders and discourage the bone crushers, most of the medication that is available to treat osteoporosis works by stopping the action of the bone crushers with the hope that the bone builders will catch up.

The reason supplements and medication are the last step of the **BONES** Lifestyle is because if you rely on them alone, they will not give you strong bones. If you do take medication for your osteopenia or osteoporosis, it is important to support the entire process of bone remodeling with a bone–healthy lifestyle by practicing balance, understanding and treating your risk factors, eating a nutritious diet, and exercising.

4

Balance Training

As you learned in Chapter 1, "The Bare Bones," a significant complication of osteoporosis is bone fracture. There is debate as to whether people with osteoporosis break bones because they fall, or if they fall because a bone broke (usually the hip). According to research, it can happen either way, depending on the location and severity of bone loss.

With that knowledge, it seems logical that you would do everything you can to prevent falls. You may become more cautious in your movement so you don't fall. You may even develop a fear of falling, and find it becomes a vicious cycle — cautious movement and a sedentary lifestyle result in a limited range of motion and a loss of functional strength. This, in turn, results in a lack of balance. Ironically, it is this caution and fear that cause many falls.

A study done by researchers from Australia and Belgium found that a fear of falling actually leads to a higher risk of falling in the future. In other studies that looked at ways to reduce falls, exercise training was repeatedly found to be the most effective intervention. As people develop functional strength and balance, confidence increases and a fear of falling decreases.

If you are at risk or have osteoporosis, you want to prevent or minimize the effects of falls. So, the first step of the BONES Lifestyle© is to improve your Balance.

The Golden Threesome: Sight, Sound, and Touch

You experience the world through your senses. With the experience of sight, sound, touch, smell, and taste, your body sends signals to your brain to tell it what's happening. The brain responds by sending signals back to your body telling it how to respond.

Imagine that you touch a hot pan. Almost instantaneously as you make contact with it, your sense of touch sends urgent signals to your brain — "HOT!" — and your brain responds by telling your muscles to pull your hand away from the pan.

The sense of touch is a key way that your body sends signals to your brain about its position and movement. It works together with your senses of sight and sound to create a feeling of balance.

Sight, sound, and touch are what I call "the golden threesome." They work together to tell your brain about your environment and your body's experience with it. If one of these senses is limited or eliminated, balance becomes difficult. Fortunately, if one of the golden three is compromised, the other two become stronger and compensate for the loss. Even if two of these senses aren't functioning, you can still develop and improve your balance. Your body has an amazing ability to overcome and compensate when faced with limitations.

Sight

Have you ever heard the saying, "What you see is what you get?" When dealing with balance I say, "What you don't see gets you!" Your eyes are constantly transmitting information to your brain, even if you are not focusing on an object. In fact, visual input accounts for about 70% of your ability to balance.

Your brain uses input from your eyes to analyze the environment. Limited vision makes it difficult to see the ground you are walking on and obstacles you may encounter. If your brain doesn't "see" what it must face, it has a difficult time responding in a timely and appropriate manner. Poor vision can also cause dizziness, which creates a type of short-circuit between your brain and body and may give you the sensation of spinning or falling.

Sound

Your ears have a built-in tool that functions like a carpenter's level or a gyroscope. It helps your brain measure stability. Fluid in the middle ear moves with your head and signals motion to your brain. This is called the vestibular system. If the fluid is compromised, by something like hearing damage or a sinus or ear infection, your brain won't get clear signals and you may feel dizzy. For some people, this dizziness occurs if they just turn their head quickly. If the fluid in your ears isn't sending a clear signal to your brain about body and head position, your brain cannot tell your body how to stabilize.

Also, as with vision, your brain uses sound to gain a sense of where you are in your environment. A loss of hearing or ringing in your ears further complicates a lack of stability by confusing your brain. Without clear signals coming through your ears from both sides, you may feel unsteady or habitually lean to one side.

Touch

Your body is constantly communicating with your brain through nerves to confirm where you are in relation to the environment and space around you. The brain then sends signals back to the muscles via the nervous system to make necessary adjustments in position, contraction, or relaxation.

The sense of touch comes from nerves located in the skin. These nerves feel pressure, motion, tension, and temperature, among other things. Working closely with the nerves in your skin are proprioceptors. Proprioceptors are key nerve centers located throughout your body that tell your brain where your body is in its space and what position your limbs and torso are in.

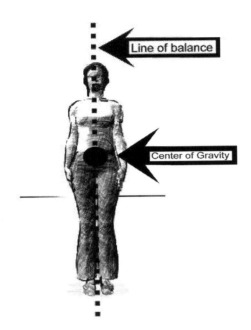

Your line of balance is like an invisible plumb line hanging down from the ceiling, perpendicular to the floor. Your line of balance should always pass through your center of gravity.

Good Posture

- *Improves balance*
- *Makes you look taller*
- *Makes you look more confident*
- *Prevents or relieves back pain*
- *Prevents headaches*
- *Improves energy*
- *Prevents injuries*
- *Improves breathing*
- *Improves circulation*
- *Improves digestion*
- *Increases self-esteem*
- *Makes you look younger*

As we age we expect some loss of hearing or vision, but many people don't realize they will also lose some of their sense of touch. Balance becomes more difficult if you lose the sense of touch in your feet or legs, or if you suffer from a stroke or illness that limits your muscular control or nerve function. Balance decreases considerably when you cannot feel full pressure on the bottoms of the feet or your proprioceptors cannot tell your brain what position your body is in.

Find Your Line of Balance, Find Your Posture

When you have good posture, balance comes naturally. Posture is physics, pure and simple. Imagine each of your body segments as separate building blocks. With each block balanced above the previous ones in a tower, your muscles and joints are free to do their job of holding you upright and moving you. If, however, the blocks are out of alignment, the joints shift, and the muscles have to put their primary job on hold to keep your tower from falling over. Think about it this way, if your shoulders are shifted forward, your upper body weight will shift forward as well. This forces your back and leg muscles to engage to keep you from falling forward onto your face.

Line of Balance

It helps to think of posture in terms of your line of balance. When standing, picture your line of balance as a plumb line hanging down from the ceiling perpendicular to the floor. Your block tower is stacked in your line of balance which will always pass through your **center of gravity**, or the center of your body's weight.

In general, your center of gravity is found at the exact center of your body. When standing, it is about one inch below your belly button. This is the point at which the top and bottom halves, the left and right halves, and the front and back halves of your body meet.

HOW TO
EVALUATE YOUR POSTURE

STANDING

To evaluate your standing posture, stand as you normally would and have someone take photos of your body from the front and from the side. Using a piece of paper or ruler as a guide, draw a straight line from the top of the picture down to the bottom. Your line on the side view picture should go straight down through your ear and on the front view picture the line should be drawn through your nose. Your pictures will look something like the ones below.

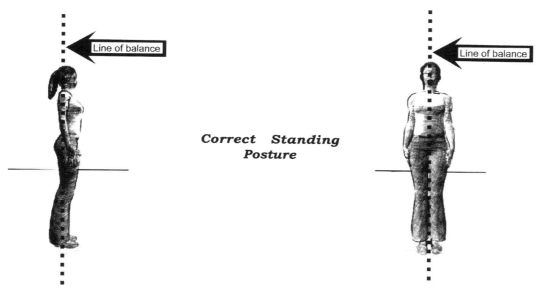

Correct Standing Posture

Evaluate your pictures to see which body parts the straight line passes through. In the front view, your torso should be aligned equally over both feet and your shoulders and hips should be level. The line will go down through your nose, the center of your chest, your belly button, and between your feet. In the side view, the center of your shoulder should be in line under the center of your earlobe. Your tailbone should point towards the floor, bringing the center of the side of your hip into alignment with your hand, which should hang directly below your shoulder. Below your hip, the outside of your knee and the prominent bone on the outside of your ankle should line up. Your toes and knees should both point towards the front.

SITTING

Next, sit on a chair with a solid seat and back (like a dining room chair). Have someone take photographs from the front and from the side. Using a guide, draw a straight line from the top of each picture down to the bottom in the same manner as you did for the standing photos — side view through your ear, front view through your nose.

When you are seated, your photo from the front view should show your head aligned over your shoulders with your chin parallel to the floor and the front of your rib cage lifted off of your hips. Does your straight line cut your face and torso in half equally between your right and left sides? Both shoulders should be at the same height and both feet should rest with equal pressure on the floor. Your knees should be at hip level.

Observe your seated posture from the side. Your earlobe should be in line with the center of your shoulder which should be slightly behind your hip. If not, a lumbar pillow or rolled towel placed behind your lower back will help you maintain this position.

Surprisingly, sitting puts more strain on your spine than standing does. A poor seated posture such as slumping or leaning forward significantly increases this stress. The safest seated position is actually a slightly reclined position with the spine maintaining its natural curves.

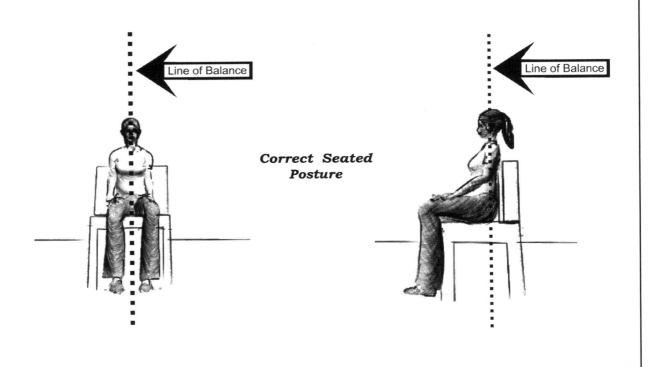

Correct Seated Posture

Line of Balance

Line of Balance

When standing, visualize your line of balance hanging down through the center of your head, through your center of gravity, and down to the floor evenly between your feet. This line is always perpendicular to the ground so when you stack your body segments along it, you place equal weight over both feet and stand balanced.

The Aligned Spine

Your spine follows your line of balance. When your spine is in correct alignment, your body's blocks will naturally stack up correctly.

Your spine is made up of 24 vertebrae plus an additional nine that are fused together to form the sacrum and coccyx (tailbone). The vertebrae are joined together to form a stretched-out letter "S" when you are standing upright, with four gentle curves that position your body directly over your legs and feet.

The bones in your spine are irregular bones connected by finger-like extensions called processes and a circular center, or centrum, to support your body's weight. The curved shape of your spine, along with the unique design of each vertebrae and proper support of your muscles, provides a strong yet flexible backbone that allows you to balance, move, rotate, and bend.

The upper section of your spine, the cervical section, attaches to and supports your head. The joint that connects the cervical vertebra to the skull is called the occipital joint. It meets the skull in the center of your head, just behind your uvula (that little dingle dangle that hangs down in the back of your throat). When your head is balanced over your spine, it rests like a golf ball propped on a tee. In this position, your chin will be parallel to the floor, exposing the gentle curves on the front and back of your neck, and your eyes will look toward the horizon where the sky meets the land.

The center curve of your spine, called the thoracic section, connects to your rib cage and provides structure for your torso. This is where most of your spine's twisting motion occurs. When you

Kyphosis

Many people assume that if a person has a rounded upper back (kyphosis) they must have osteoporosis. It is true that osteoporosis can cause a curved spine because vertebral compression fractures typically occur at the front of a vertebra. This forms a wedge shape that causes the spine to tilt forward, into a dowager's hump. It puts tremendous strain on the muscles, and causes severe pain.

But it is possible to have a rounded upper back without vertebral fractures. Many cases of kyphosis are actually a result of poor posture and muscle imbalance. If you don't align your spine, or the upper back muscles are weaker than the chest muscles, the chest will pull the shoulders forward, rounding the upper back. This is also quite painful. Whatever the cause, kyphosis can be helped with posture exercises.

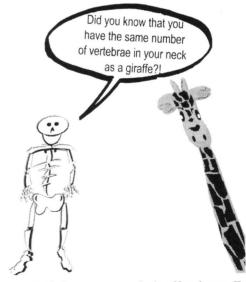

Both humans and giraffes have 7 bones in their necks.

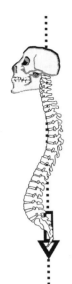

When your head is balanced over your spine with normal curvature, the line of balance goes through the center of the top of your head and through the center of your sacrum.

twist your torso, your rib cage is actually rotating over your hips. Each vertebra rotates until it catches the finger-like projections on the vertebra above it. This creates a spiralling motion that twists the spine like a barber pole.

The lower curve of your spine, called the lumbar section, has the largest vertebrae and bears most of your body's weight. Located at the bottom of the lumbar section are the sacrum and coccyx which form a triangle pointing down toward the floor like an arrowhead. I call this the "sacral arrow." The point of this arrow is also what people refer to as the tailbone. The arrow may point toward the floor, at an angle toward the front, or at an angle toward the back.

Attached to the sacrum, at the base of your spine is your pelvis. It is shaped like a bowl. Imagine it as a bowl of pancake batter. When your tailbone, or "sacral arrow," is pointed toward the floor, your pelvis "bowl" is flat as if it were set on a counter. This is called a neutral pelvis position. When you tilt the pelvis forward, pointing your

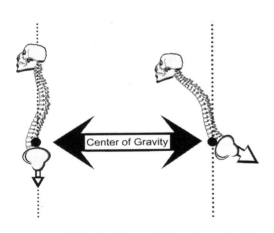

Center of Gravity

Your pelvis is shaped like a bowl with the center of gravity sitting just above it. When standing upright, your pelvic bowl should be tilted as if it is sitting flat on the counter so the "sacral arrow" is pointing down toward the floor. When you squat, your pelvis tips forward as if you are pouring out the pancake batter and your "sacral arrow" points at an angle behind you.

Bowling Anyone?

Your head is roughly the same weight as a bowling ball (about 10 lbs.). When balanced over your spine, it does not add strain to your neck muscles. However, for every inch that your head moves in front of your line of balance, your neck muscles will have to hold up the weight equivalent to 10 times the distance from the line. If you tip your head forward one inch, your head will feel like 10 X 1 or 10 pounds of strain to your neck. If you tip your head forward two inches to look down at the ground, the muscles in your neck must hold up 10 X 2 or 20 pounds! In this position, your neck and back muscles have to work overtime just to keep your head on. The muscles don't like this extra work, so if you look down at the ground too much, they will rebel by going into spasm and causing back pain, shoulder pain, neck pain, and headaches. This habit can also lead to kyphosis, a condition where the upper back rounds forward creating a humpback appearance.

"arrow" behind you at an angle, it is as if you are pouring the pancake batter out onto the griddle. If you don't also bring your chest forward when you tip your pelvis forward, you will exaggerate the curve of your lower back.

In front of your spine, just above your pelvic bowl, your center of gravity defines your balance. This center of gravity is where your body weight is concentrated. Because your center of gravity changes slightly when you move or lift an object, it's not always easy to feel it. Many people like to visualize a brightly colored ball or an anchor sitting at this point to bring the mind and body together. Remember, your line of balance must go through your center of gravity for you to be balanced.

When you stand, your spine should be in line over your pelvis, which in turn should be balanced over both legs so your weight is evenly distributed between your feet. You should be able to feel the balls of your big toes, the balls of your little toes and your heels all in contact with the floor, with even pressure over each of them. This is known as the tripod of the foot. If you feel more pressure forward or back or to one side, it means your center of gravity is shifted and your block tower is out of alignment. The spine is designed to align the body directly over the feet, and the feet are designed to support the body.

Counterbalance

Good posture is not just about standing up straight. It's also about letting the correct muscles do their job. Your body will function at its best when you keep your line of balance in mind for all positions and movements – walking, bending, sitting, kneeling, and even lying down. Remember, your line of balance always hangs straight down from the ceiling through your center of gravity and perpendicular to the floor. If you shift your body's center of gravity to one side of your line (right, left, front, back, or diagonally), something must provide resistance so you don't fall over.

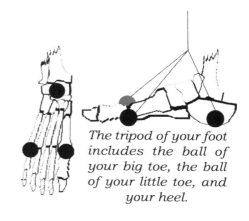

The tripod of your foot includes the ball of your big toe, the ball of your little toe, and your heel.

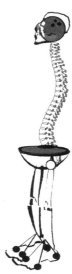

Put the posture picture together and you've got a bowling ball balanced over a bowl of pancake batter which is sitting level over two tripods.

You can use opposing muscles to hold your body up, until the weight shifts too far, at which point you must adjust the rest of your body in some way to keep from falling. You can move your body under the shifted weight as you do when you walk, or you can reach something toward the opposite side of your line of balance.

Shifting another body part in the opposite direction — to the opposite side of your line of balance — is called **counterbalance**. For example, if you push your hips back to sit in a chair, more of your weight is behind your line of balance. To stay relaxed and remain stable, you can add counterbalance by bringing your chest, shoulders, and arms in front of your line of balance.

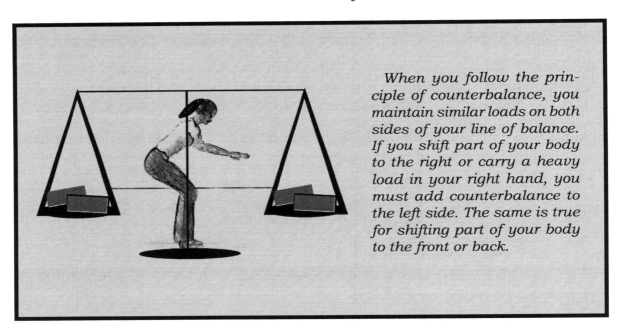

When you follow the principle of counterbalance, you maintain similar loads on both sides of your line of balance. If you shift part of your body to the right or carry a heavy load in your right hand, you must add counterbalance to the left side. The same is true for shifting part of your body to the front or back.

To understand counterbalance, think of a pan scale. In a pan scale, the dish or pan on one side is weighted with a known weight and the opposite dish is loaded to equalize the scale. When your body has the same load on both sides of the line of balance, the workload is distributed to the bones, muscles, and joints that are designed for the work, freeing up the rest of the body (including your internal organs) to do their job.

HOW TO
EVALUATE YOUR BALANCE

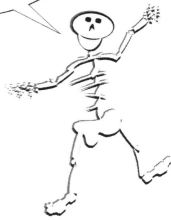

If you have advanced osteoporosis, a current fracture, or other physical limitations, be sure to clear all exercises with your physician or physical therapist before beginning.

To increase confidence in your movement and prevent unwanted falls, your osteoporosis program (or any exercise program, for that matter) should begin with posture and balance training. The exercises in this chapter are designed to strengthen your core, improve your body mechanics, and decrease strain on your back.

SINGLE LEG BALANCE

Hold onto a chair or table and lift one foot off the floor for 5 to 10 seconds. If you are very unsteady, have someone stand near you. If you can stand on one foot and balance successfully, try letting go of the chair or table.

Now, put both feet down and think about your shoulders and neck — notice how they feel. Did they tense up? Did your shoulders ride up near your ears or round forward as you tried to balance? What were you thinking about when your foot was lifted? Did you feel wobbly? Did you hold your breath? Try the exercise again and notice your mind's and body's reactions.

Most people approach balance as something to conquer. If I asked you to speak your thoughts out loud while you stood on one foot, I'd likely hear something like, "If I really concentrate on staying still, then I can balance. I'm staying still. . . staying still. . . lifting my leg. . . I don't want to fall. . . I will balance. . . I used to be able to do this. . . what is wrong with me?" If your self-talk sounds anything like this, you will end up teetering, stepping down and feeling frustrated.

This self-talk and your response to balancing on one foot are all normal responses as your brain tries to figure out where your body is in space and how to keep you stable. But by tensing your upper body, you change your posture. If you lean to one side or bend forward to prevent falling, you are shifting your center of gravity and actually throwing your body out of balance even more. This puts more strain on your muscles as they try to hold you up.

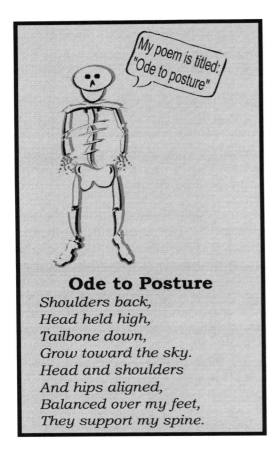

Ode to Posture

Shoulders back,
Head held high,
Tailbone down,
Grow toward the sky.
Head and shoulders
And hips aligned,
Balanced over my feet,
They support my spine.

Mind Over Body, Body Over Mind

Posture is closely related to your emotional state. Low self-esteem, anxiety, or depression can all lead to poor posture. But on the flip side, good posture often promotes a sense of wellness. If you tend to hunch your back, consider possible psychological causes. Are you tall or big-chested? Were you teased as a child and developed a pose that allowed you to hide? Do you feel insecure when you are around other people? Are you a worrier?

When you find yourself slouching or looking at the ground, take a moment to evaluate your emotional state. If you recognize a connection, acknowledge it. Then when you find yourself slouching, visualize your line of balance and center of gravity, stack your tower of blocks, and recite this poem: "Shoulders back, head held high, tailbone down, grow toward the sky. Head and shoulders and hips aligned, balanced over my feet, they support my spine." Look out to the horizon, hold your head up, and believe in yourself.

No matter your age, you can improve your quality of movement by focusing on balance. Unfortunately, as with all other fitness components, if you don't use it, you'll lose it. You may have been able to stand on a ball and juggle three eggs when you were 10 years old, but if you haven't kept practicing, you won't be able to do that now! The good news is that with training, you can recover some of the innate balance you had as a child.

Balance is a bit contradictory, because you are most balanced and steady when you let go and relax. Remember when you were young and could hop effortlessly across the rocks in a creek? You didn't worry about slipping or falling. You believed you could do it because you had no reason not to believe. You let go of inhibitions and skimmed over the creek. But if your mom yelled, "Be careful! Don't fall!"? You may have paused and let fear take hold. Once that fear got ahold of you, you'd tense up, change your posture, focus on the next foot that was lifting or the rock you were stepping to. You would either make it across shaking, or fall right into the creek!

Fear of falling is a big reason you may adopt a sedentary lifestyle. Maybe you grew up with fear, have had a bad fall, or just feel that you are less stable than you used to be. Poor vision, inner ear imbalances, illness, injuries, and certain medications may make you dizzy or unsteady so you don't want to take any risks. Your sedentary lifestyle may be a defensive response to fear. This is understandable, but it may put you in more peril — not less. A lack of mobility weakens muscles, decreases reflexes, and increases the risk of falls.

Balance requires coordination between your mind and body. It is not something you can force, rather it is something you allow to happen. You must understand the principles behind balance and believe you can do it. Remember your pelvic bowl and center of gravity? When shifting your weight to one foot, the only way you will be able to balance over that single foot is if you have good posture and you shift your center of gravity over the standing foot. This requires confidence be-

> Shift your center of gravity

When shifting your weight to one foot, start with good posture then shift your center of gravity over the standing foot. Your belly button will be in line with the bow of your shoelace and your upper body will shift with your center of gravity.

Have fun with balance: *Press one side of your body against a wall — the outside of one foot, knee, hip, and shoulder. With that side still pressed against the wall, try to lift the other foot off the floor. Can you do it? If you can, you are either extremely talented or cheating!!!! You should not be able to get your foot off the floor for any more than a brief second. This is because with the wall against the side of your body, your center of gravity can't shift over the standing leg to balance and support your body. Unless you shift your center over your base of support, you cannot maintain balance. This is an example of functional movement. You may not realize that you shift your center of gravity over your base of support every time you step, but you do.*

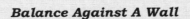

Balance Against A Wall

cause the shift is actually farther over than you think, but if you don't get your weight over that foot, you will not be able to maintain your balance and will have to step back down to the floor.

Thoracic Breathing

Everybody knows you have to breathe but it's amazing how many people hold their breath when they concentrate on balancing. Breathing is an essential component of exercise. Not only does it nourish the blood with oxygen and expel stale air, but did you know that your balance is at its best as you exhale? If done correctly, your breathing will help you engage your core muscles and stabilize your spine so you are relaxed and balanced in any position.

Thoracic breathing emphasizes the lower part of the lungs, located in front of the thoracic region of the spine. The thoracic vertebrae are in the center section of your spine – the area surrounded by your rib cage. Most people use only a portion of their lung capacity when breathing. But by allowing your rib cage to expand and contract with each breath, thoracic breathing allows the breath to completely fill your lungs. You may also hear this breathing technique called diaphragm, lateral, or three-dimensional breathing.

The goal of thoracic breathing is to draw air in three-dimensionally, filling your lungs to the front, sides, and back. You should feel the air fall into the lower portion of your lungs, allowing for deep, stabilizing breaths.

Interestingly, you fill your lungs with air by relaxing. The breathing cycle begins with an exhale. This is where the effort occurs. By engaging your deep core muscles on the exhale, you push all the old, stale air up and out of your lungs. Then, when your lungs have room for new, fresh air, simply relax your abdominal and chest muscles and let the diaphragm muscle draw in new air like a vacuum.

HOW TO

THORACIC BREATHING EXERCISE

This breathing technique may be difficult at first if you are like most people who only breath in the upper third of their lungs, but with practice it will become second nature. It helps to imagine that your torso is shaped like a vase with a full round base at the bottom of your lungs down into your abdominal cavity and a thin neck extending through the upper rib cage into your neck.

Wrap a towel behind your back around the lower part of your rib cage, holding it in front with one end of the towel in each hand. Begin your breath with an exhale, pushing the air out through your mouth. Try to push all the air out by flattening your belly toward your spine. Imagine that your vase is full of water and you are pushing the water up and out of the top by squeezing the bottom of the vase. Feel your back and sides pull away from the towel as you exhale.

Once all the old air is out of your lungs, relax your abdominal muscles and allow new air to come in through your nose. Feel your back and sides press outward against the towel. Your belly will also expand forward, but try not to move the upper part of your ribs or your shoulders. As the new air comes in, it will fill the vase as if it were a steady stream of water pouring into the bottom first then filling the neck of the vase at the very end of your inhale. With each inhale, focus on the expansion of your back and sides against the towel.

Practice this technique daily. It's a great exercise to do when you get out of the shower since you already have a towel in your hands.

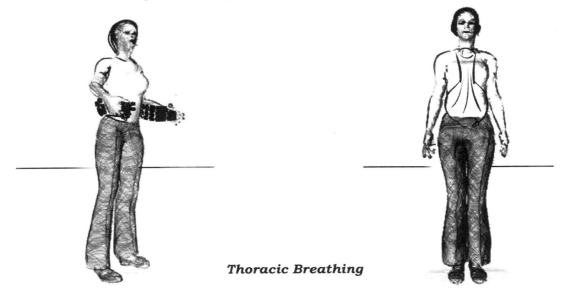

Thoracic Breathing

HOW TO
BALANCE EXERCISES

POSTURE EXERCISE

To check your posture and find your line of balance, do this simple exercise. Stand with your feet hip-width apart and your weight evenly spread over the tripods of each foot. Lift your arms out to the sides and rotate your palms toward the sky. Bend your knees slightly and tilt your pelvis into a neutral position — tailbone pointed to the floor, belly button pulled in towards the spine, rear end relaxed. Feel your shoulder blades pull slightly back and down towards the floor as the center of your chest lifts to the sky. Expose the gentle curve of your neck and look towards the horizon. In this position, you have good posture. Rotate your palms to face forward and slowly lower your hands down to your sides without changing anything else. This is how you should maintain your spinal alignment throughout the day. Anytime you need a posture check, repeat this exercise.

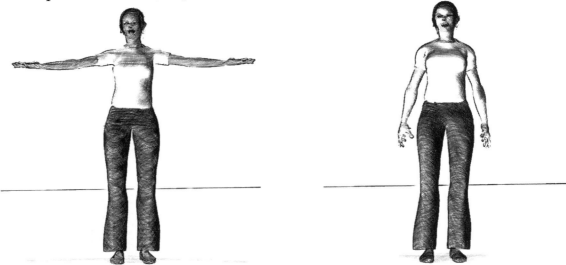

Posture Check

CENTER OF GRAVITY BALANCE

Stand by your chair or table again. This time, relax and breathe full smooth thoracic breaths into the base of your vase. Exhale for 6 seconds, pushing all the stale air out. Then, inhale for 4 seconds, expanding your rib cage to the front, back, and sides. Feel the lower part of your ribs open out and lift up off the hips as the space between your ribs and hips gets longer.

Check your posture and focus on your body's center of gravity – about an inch below your belly button in the center of your body. Remember, this is where the right and left sides of your body come together, the upper and lower halves, and the front and back. Visualize your block tower — your head should be aligned over your shoulders, which are over your pelvis, which is over your ankles. Your knees are a slightly bent link in line with both your pelvis and ankles. Got all that? Now you are ready to progress.

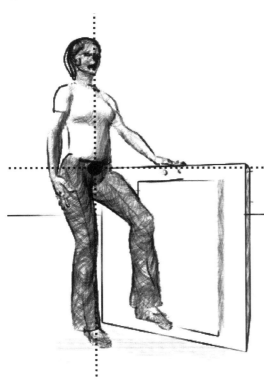

Center Of Gravity Balance

Once your body is aligned with your line of balance, maintain that position and shift your center of gravity over one foot. Lift the other heel off the floor. As you do this, realign your tower of blocks over the standing foot (your base of support). Resist that little voice inside your head that tells you to focus on the foot you are lifting. Instead, keep your mind on your center of gravity, stand tall, and relax your shoulders. Press down on the table if needed.

Feel your block tower stacked over the tri-pod of the standing foot and keep your mind focused on the center of your body, balanced over your one-footed base. Point your sacral arrow toward the floor to scoop your pelvis into a neutral position and lift the other foot all the way off the floor. As you do this, you will feel your belly button pull back toward your spine.

Take your time, move slowly and fluidly and release any muscle tension as it creeps in. If you need to put your foot down, do so, take another deep full breath and start again. The floor is always just a step away so

Confidence is key. Believe that you can balance because you can. Some people use assistance from a wall, countertop, cane, or walker. That is fine. Start simply and gradually increase the challenge. Spend time each day playing with physics and training your body to stabilize itself. You will be thrilled with the results!

don't panic if you wobble a little — just put your foot down, then start again.

To help you keep your focus, stare at a stationary point on the floor about 5 to 10 feet ahead of you — far enough out that you keep your chin up, your neck gently curved and your spine aligned. Balance on one foot for 5 to 10 seconds then touch back down. If you're feeling unsteady, use a table or wall for support, gradually releasing your hold to one finger, then none as you feel more centered and balanced.

> *The following additional challenges should only be added after you are totally stable with the basic work and are ready for a greater challenge. Done too early, the challenge exercises may lead to falls or injury.*

POSTURE PLUS

Once you become more adept at aligning your spine while standing, try this exercise. Place a small ball or cup of water in each hand. Lift your arms out to the sides, palms rotated toward the sky, hands open so the balls or cups are balanced on the center of your palms. As you balance the balls or cups on your palms, the center of your body will respond with greater balance too because you subconsciously engage your core muscles whenever you balance something on your hands or head. Now try lifting one foot and stepping to the side or front. Feel your center of gravity shift, but don't let your cups spill or your balls fall!

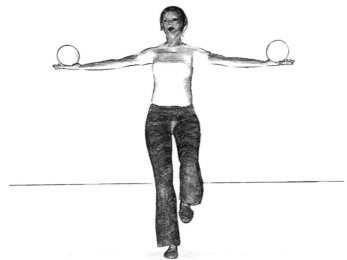

Balance With Balls

As you are developing your balance, you may notice that your foot and ankle move or your upper body sways when you stand on one foot. This is because a balanced body is never perfectly still. Since the earth is moving in space, there is a circular swaying motion that occurs in the body all the time — you simply become more aware of this when you are challenging your balance. Allow your weight to shift slightly in a circular motion through the "tripod" of the foot — the ball of the big toe, the ball of the little toe and the heel. This subtle weight shift puts pressure on different nerves in your foot which is one way your body and brain communicate with each other. As you become aware of this subtle shifting of weight and the adjustments your body makes to tell your brain where it is in space, you will be more comfortable balancing.

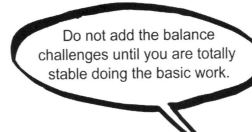

Do not add the balance challenges until you are totally stable doing the basic work.

BALANCE CHALLENGE

Once you can stand relaxed on one foot for at least 30 seconds, start moving your arms overhead or in circles. You may enjoy tossing a ball from one hand to the other. When you add movement to the rest of your body, you increase the challenge to your core muscles and your balancing leg.

Next, try to keep one foot lifted while you hold your arms still and straighten the lifted leg out to the front, then bring it back to the center. Straighten it out to the side, then bring it back to center. Straighten it behind your torso, and bring it back to the center.

Finally, draw some smooth sideways figure eights (an infinity sign) out in front of your body with your arms and/ or legs. If you keep your mind focused on your center of gravity, you should be able to move both arms and the lifted leg in any pattern and stay steady. Practice this next to a counter or table so you can hold on if needed. As your balance improves, you won't need as much assistance.

Once you feel steady and can easily repeat these challenges without assistance, practice with your eyes closed. Always keep your moves fluid and controlled and keep your spine aligned — do not use momentum to move and don't arch or round your back.

Why Do People Fall?

Let's face it, falling stinks! In an ideal world, we would prevent all falls, but unfortunately, that is not possible. Age doesn't matter. People fall. A fall may occur for any number of reasons but there are some common causes:

- Disorientation or confusion
- Startle reflex
- Rushing
- Fear or anxiety
- Feeling overextended or distracted
- Dizziness or vertigo
- Sinus problems
- Inner ear imbalance
- Hearing difficulties
- Vision difficulties
- Shortened stride/shuffle step
- Gait change due to stroke or illness
- Joint pain
- Unsteady gait
- Limited range of motion
- Low blood pressure
- Low blood sugar
- Loss of sensation in feet or legs
- Weak muscles
- Fatigue
- Poor balance
- Medications
- Alcohol

If you have fragile bones due to osteoporosis, falls become more hazardous. It is important to take precautions to prevent falling. The most important precaution is what you've learned in this chapter — improve your posture and balance.

As you walk, slow down, look out ahead, and scan the room on both sides and in front of you for any possible obstacles. Use your peripheral vision to warn you of moving obstacles, and be certain that you have a firm footing before you shift your body weight onto the new foot. Additional skill development to help prevent falls is in the Exercise chapter (Chapter 7).

> *About 50% of all people age 80 and older fall at least once a year.*

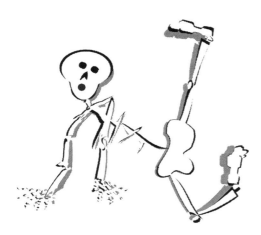

Falls happen when we least expect them.

HOW TO
AVOID FALLS

1. Lift your foot all the way up off the ground when you take a step.
2. Change medications if yours is causing dizziness.
3. Use hearing aids if you have difficulty hearing.
4. Treat sinus congestion with saline washes, nasal spray, or medication.
5. Wear glasses if you need them.
6. Slow down and take your time.
7. Use a cane, walking stick, or walker if you feel unsteady or will be walking on uneven surfaces.
8. Stand near a counter or chair when practicing balance exercises.
9. Avoid carrying heavy loads up or down stairs or on hills.
10. Avoid carrying large items in front of you so you can't see your feet.
11. Make sure your home is well lit and use nightlights.
12. Wear non-skid shoes and slippers.
13. Place handrails in your bathroom, bedroom, hallway, and front walkway. Make sure stairs have secure handrails.
14. Tape throw rugs securely to the floor or get rid of them.
15. Pick up clutter.
16. Put bells on your pets so you know where they are.
17. Put a traction mat in your bathtub or shower so it is less slippery.

Physics of Falling

It is important to understand the physics of falling. The first step in fall prevention is to be aware of what causes you to lose your balance and secondly, what happens when you do. To date, no scientific studies that I know of have been done to see how people land when pushed or tripped from behind, although a day in a preschool classroom might shed some light on the subject. But some experiments have been done with willing participants who used pads to break their falls.

What these studies found is that if you turn quickly and catch your foot, you will probably fall to the side or to the back.

If you are startled, you are most likely to fall to the back or side since the startle reflex causes people to jump or lean away from the input. This is a common cause of falling for older people who are losing their sense of hearing or sight.

When someone trips or unexpectedly steps down off a curb or step, they typically fall forward. This is why you must be careful if you are on the top step of a staircase. Likewise, if you catch your toe on a rug, step, or curb when you are walking forward, you will likely fall forward. But if you are stepping to the side or back and catch your foot you will probably fall in the direction you were stepping because momentum will carry you over.

Walking sideways on a hill causes some people to fall downhill but if they overcompensate, they may fall into the uphill side. Walking uphill causes some people to fall backwards, and walking downhill causes some people to fall forward. This is more likely if they are walking slowly.

If you slip or faint when you are walking at a brisk pace, you will probably fall forward. If you are moving slowly and slip or faint, you are more likely to fall to the side or to the back.

Slipping on the ice or a slick floor will cause you to fall forward if you are moving fast, or to the back if you are moving slowly.

If Ya Gotta Fall, Do It Right!

One day I was walking backwards on a sidewalk, talking to a friend. At the end of our conversation, I intended to spin around to continue on my way — facing the direction I was going. But I had made the mistake of not scanning my path before turning to walk backwards, and as we walked, I had backed right up to a park bench that was in the path. As I spun around, my leg caught the bench and stopped the lower half of my body while the momentum of moving and spinning kept pulling my upper half forward. There was no stopping it! That moment after I knew I'd lost my balance and before I landed on the ground seemed to last forever. My panic instincts took over. I stuck out my hands and tensed my whole body, landing awkwardly on my hands and knees. It probably hurt even more because I knew it could have been prevented had I slowed down and previewed my environment.

HOW TO

FALL

Ideally, you will be able to prevent a fall by staying focused and aware of your environment, but what should you do if you catch your foot on the edge of a curb (or your leg on the edge of a park bench!) and can't get it back under you to stop a fall? There is actually a good way to fall – one that decreases your chances of injury. Gymnasts, martial artists, and other athletes are taught to fall correctly because their coaches know they run a high risk of hitting the ground. One of the keys to successful falling is to let the fall happen and go with it. Bring your arms in close to your body, bend your knees to lower your center of gravity, and roll to your side.

In contrast to my messy sprawl onto the sidewalk, I've seen people lose their balance the right way. One day a friend of mine was walking across the room towards me. I saw her center of gravity shift and knew she wasn't going to be able to get her foot underneath her. She has multiple sclerosis, a neurological condition that can lead to a loss of muscle control, so for her, falls are common. No one was close to her, and I was too far away to stop the fall.

But as I ran towards her, I witnessed beauty in motion. She had felt her balance shift and knew she was going to fall. Instead of fighting it as I had, she gracefully swooned to the floor like a feather. I was so impressed by her poise that I asked her what she was thinking as she fell. She joked that she'd had a lot of practice but then shared this wonderful advice: "It's like turning in the direction of the skid when your car is slipping on ice," she said. "Once you know you're skidding, you have to just ride it out." When you know you can't stop a fall, your best bet is to go with it. Try to relax and let the momentum carry you through so you can roll as smoothly as possible. Rolling is easier on your bones because it spreads the impact over multiple body parts instead of focusing it all on your hands, knees, shoulder, or hip.

PRACTICE MAKES PERFECT

Do not practice falling if you have severe (advanced) osteoporosis, a current fracture, or any other injuries or limitations! *Always follow safety guidelines when exercising: have someone nearby who can assist you as needed, move within your range and ability, use appropriate tools for assistance (pillows, cane, walker, straps, etc.)*

If you are strong enough, it's not a bad idea to practice falling in a safe environment so your muscles and brain have some memory of the experience if you start to fall. Muscle memory is a valuable benefit of exercise. When your body moves, your brain and body develop an "experience record" that flows through a pathway of nerves that communicate with your muscles. This record can be replayed the next time your body moves that way so the movement comes more easily. With each successive experience, the memory becomes clearer so your brain can direct your body more quickly and with less conscious thought.

A good place to practice falling is on your bed. Have someone available to assist you when you practice this exercise. Sit on your bed, with one arm tucked in close to your body. Relax and lean toward that side, allowing yourself to roll from your hip to your shoulder. Keep your neck stable so your head doesn't hit hard on the bed. Practice rolling to the same side several times then try rolling to the other side and then to your back. Bring your knees in towards your chest as you roll. This will assist with the rolling and will help you control your "fall" by contracting your core muscles.

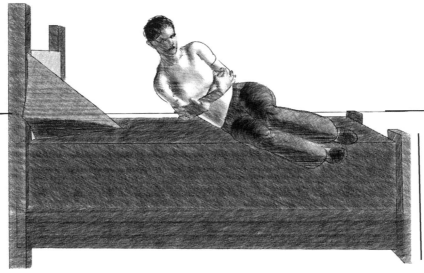

Practice Fall

Osteoporosis Tests

When it comes to diagnosing and treating osteoporosis, we are fortunate to have a plethora of technological advances in our favor. However, when we have so many options to choose from, it can be easy to forget about good ol' common sense. We hear about the horrors of diseases like osteoporosis and our fear drives us to jump before we look.

Don't misunderstand me. Osteoporosis is a devastating condition, and it's prevalence is a serious concern for our medical system and for us as individuals. If I didn't believe that, I wouldn't have written this book.

But I also wrote this book to help you understand exactly what is happening to your bones. I often have clients contact me in tears because they just received the grave diagnosis of *osteoporosis*. Just one word and they picture their active lifestyle cut short. No more playing tennis or skiing. No more afternoons in the park with their kids, grandkids, or pets. No more horseback rides on the beach. Boom! One word and they see themselves struggling with a walker.

Before you condemn yourself to the couch, you must know the why's and how's of your diagnosis. Education is your best friend when it comes to your health. With knowledge you are equipped to make wise decisions. So this book wouldn't be complete without a chapter explaining the O of the BONES Lifestyle© — Osteoporosis Tests.

HOW TO
KNOW YOUR RISK FACTORS

Osteoporosis can strike anyone at any age but some people have a greater chance of getting it. Age is the number one determinate of risk. The older you are, the more likely it is that you've lost some bone. But risks are also cumulative — the more risk factors you have, the greater your chances are of losing bone.

Place a check mark next to the risk factors you have or may have. If you have multiple risk factors, you should take steps to preserve your bone mineral density, including having a bone mineral density test done to determine your current bone mineral density.

RISK FACTORS FOR OSTEOPOROSIS

__ Age
__ Family history of osteoporosis, or fractures of spine or hip
__ Very thin or very tall build
__ Inactivity
__ History of smoking
__ Female
__ Post-menopausal
__ Caucasian or Asian descent
__ Low vitamin D intake or minimal exposure to sunlight
__ Low calcium intake
__ Personal history of anorexia nervosa or bulimia
__ Chronic illnesses such as type 1 diabetes, liver or kidney disease, or hyperthyroidism
__ Chronic use of corticosteroids, such as prednisone (inhalation steroids taken in low to moderate doses for long-term treatment of asthma do not seem to increase the risk of osteoporosis and fractures)
__ Difficulty absorbing nutrients due to a gastrointestinal illness, surgically removed gall bladder, excessive dieting, or long-term use of laxatives, antacids, or acid blockers
__ Deficiencies in estrogen or testosterone
__ Chemotherapy treatment
__ Rheumatoid arthritis or juvenile rheumatoid arthritis
__ Overactive or underactive parathyroid or thyroid gland and use of thyroid hormone
__ Periods of immobilization or time spent in space at zero gravity
__ Late onset of menstrual cycle or early menopause

Check your risk factors

___ Lengthy bouts with depression and treatment with SSRIs (selective serotonin reuptake inhibitors)
___ Use of anti-seizure medications such as Dilantin
___ Drinking excessive caffeine or alcohol
___ Eating a very high protein or high sodium diet
___ Blonde or redhead with fair skin
___ Premature gray hair

Multiple risk factors indicate a greater potential for fracture, but don't fret if you have several of them. It doesn't mean you are destined to break a hip. What it does mean is that you should evaluate your lifestyle and make any necessary changes to decrease your risks.

Begin by discussing your situation and risk factors with your doctor. Ask for a bone mineral density scan to evaluate your current BMD. (This is the **O** of the **BONES** Lifestyle.) Then make sure you read the rest of this book to learn how you can incorporate the **BONES** Lifestyle into your life.

Although postmenopausal women who are Caucasian or Asian are usually considered at higher risk of developing osteoporosis, it occurs in all racial groups and in both sexes.

As many as 49% of Mexican-American women 50 years of age or older have low bone mineral density.

Asian-American women have less chance of sustaining a hip fracture than Caucasian women, but the rate of vertebral fractures is about equal in these two races.

African-American women typically have stronger bones than other races, but about 10 percent of African-American women over 50 still have osteoporosis and an additional 30 percent have low bone mineral density. Up to 95 percent of fractures experienced by African-American women over age 64 are related to osteoporosis.

About one in eight men will experience an osteoporotic fracture and one-third of all hip fractures experienced by men are related to osteoporosis. Men over age 70 are at highest risk. Osteoporosis in males is typically related to an illness, long-term steroid therapy, high alcohol consumption, or low physical activity.

Osteoporosis Indicators

Does it seem that you've shrunk in height over the years? Some loss of height is normal and is often due to weak torso muscles. But if your height has dropped significantly since your twenties, there is a chance it could be due to osteoporosis. A simple test you can do to tell if you've lost height is to measure your arm span from fingertip to fingertip. On average, this distance is equal to your height at the peak of your growth curve, around your mid-20s. If there is a significant difference between this measurement and your current height, your height loss may be due to osteoporosis. But even if you have lost some height, don't panic. Loss of height isn't a sure diagnosis of osteoporosis, it's just a possible side effect.

There are a number of indicators of bone loss. Take time to consider side effects and indicators you might have.

Kyphosis, or rounding of the upper back, may be a sign that you've experienced vertebral fractures. It can be a simple case of weak muscles. But if you have sustained a number of compression fractures in your vertebrae, the vertebrae will tilt forward, and your upper back may form a rounded humpback, also known as a dowager's hump.

Your dentist may see periodontal disease or signs of bone loss in your jaw on your dental x-rays. This may indicate bone loss in other parts of your body as well.

Bone loss and muscle mass often go hand in hand. If you've lost significant muscle mass throughout your body, you may have also lost some bone mass. Studies show a correlation between hand grip strength, strength of the upper arm, and bone mineral density in the forearm. There is also a correlation between strength of the thigh muscles, and bones in the hip and spine.

Finally, bone growth is similar to the growth of your fingernails, toenails, and hair. Changes in the health of your nails or hair may signify an imbalance in your body. For example, weak or

> *At peak bone mineral density, most people's arm span (measured from fingertip to fingertip with arms spread out to the sides) is equal to their height. There are some exceptions to this rule but if your height is significantly less than the length of your arm span, you may be losing height.*

brittle nails or prematurely gray hair can be an indicator of potential osteoporosis.

These side effects are indicators that something may be amiss in your bone remodeling cycle, but none of them is a definitive diagnosis of osteoporosis. The only absolute way to know if you have osteoporosis is to sustain a fragility fracture — a fracture that occurs after a minimal trauma.

Keep in mind that not all fractures that occur in adulthood are fragility fractures. If you've sustained one or more fractures in your lifetime, it does not mean you have osteoporosis. However your risk may be higher if you've had fractures that occurred without much force or impact, or you have one or more of the side effects listed above. Discuss your risk factors and the possibility of a bone mineral density test with your doctor. If your bone mineral density is low, you will want to shift your BONES Lifestyle into high gear.

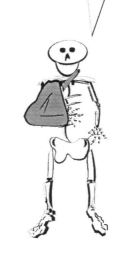

Half of all postmenopausal women will have an osteoporosis-related fracture during their lifetime.

Osteoporosis Tests

Since most of us don't want to wait until a bone breaks to find out that we have osteoporosis, medical scientists have come up with a way to measure bone mineral density. Like height loss, kyphosis, periodontal disease, and decreased muscle mass, bone mineral density is an estimate of bone strength.

Bone densitometry is one method for measuring bone mineral density. It is non-intrusive, requires a minimal time commitment, and delivers a very low dose of radiation, making it safe and convenient. It is also much less painful than the "bone-breaking method" described above.

Currently, the National Osteoporosis Foundation (NOF) recommends bone mineral density testing for all women over age 65 and for women under the age of 65 who have one or more risk factors for osteoporosis, not including menopause. If your doctor prescribes drug therapy for osteoporosis, he/she will probably recommend follow-up bone mineral density scans to monitor your rate of bone mineral loss and your response to the medication.

Most doctors start their analysis with a bone mineral density test, but if your doctor is concerned about your risk of fracture, he/she may recommend additional tests. Lab tests to measure the amount of collagen and calcium in a urine sample or the amount of calcium, phosphorus, and estrogen in a blood sample will give your doctor an idea about how your bones are remodeling. A blood test cannot diagnose osteoporosis, it can only signal potential problems that may indicate bone loss. If your doctor suspects an underlying illness may be leading to your low bone mineral density, he may also order blood or urine samples for further analysis.

Dual–energy x–ray absorptiometry (DEXA) is currently the bone densitometry test of choice for most doctors because it is accurate and widely available. To date, bone mineral density measured at the **femoral neck** (at the top of the thigh bone) by DEXA is the best predictor of hip fracture and is comparable to forearm measurements for predicting fractures at other sites. DEXA measures the bone in planes and has low spatial resolution so it cannot distinguish between trabecular bone and cortical bone, nor can it identify bone geometry. It only measures the mineral density of the bone in specific areas. A DEXA test alone cannot provide an absolute diagnosis of osteoporosis. It can only predict risk.

While the DEXA test is the most commonly prescribed, there are other ways to measure your bone mineral density. The following tests all measure bone mineral density plus content and tell you how stiff the bone is: Radiographic Absorptiometry (RA), Single Energy X–ray Absorptiometry (SXA), Peripheral Dual–energy X–ray Absorptiometry (PDXA) and Peripheral Quantitative Computed Tomography (pQCT).

Quantitative Ultrasonography (QUS), or ultrasound, provides a different measurement of bone strength. It measures total bone strength – bone

For women, a difference in measurements of bone mineral density between sites is typically more pronounced in the years just following menopause. During these years, it is common for density to be normal at one site and low at another. The trabecular (spongy) bone tissue shows the first signs of breakdown because it has more surface area. Remember, bone remodeling occurs on the surface of the bones. Because vertebrae have a higher percentage of trabecular tissue than other bones, the spine usually has greater turnover and is often the first site to show signs of decreased bone mineral density.

mineral density (stiffness) and bone flexibility (the ability of bone to give with impact), which is important for fracture prevention. As you learned in Chapter 1, total bone strength is actually a better predictor of fracture, but ultrasound is currently limited in its accuracy and ability to measure key sites such as the hip and spine. In the future, ultrasound may prove more reliable than DEXA for determining bone strength.

You must consider all the sites when you look at your scores because the scores are mostly site specific. The most common tests give results for your spine and femoral neck at the hip. Be sure you understand the meaning of the scores for both of these areas. Ask your doctor if you have questions.

Peripheral tests that are measured at your wrist, finger, or heel are not an accurate predictor of bone mineral density in your femoral neck (hip) or spine. These sites typically have a higher bone mineral density because your hands and heels are subjected to different stresses daily as you move about. If you have one of these tests and the results are low, you may want to follow up with a DEXA scan of your hip and spine.

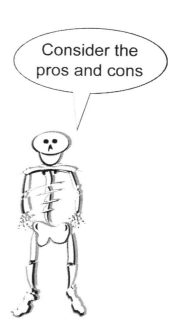

Consider the pros and cons

Also keep in mind that some physical characteristics affect the scans. For example, spinal degeneration can cause a false positive on a DEXA scan and report a higher T-score when the bone is actually less dense. If you have experienced arthritic changes in your spine (which is common among elderly patients), the bone mineral density there may appear to be higher than it actually is. In this case you would want to compare these scores to your bone mineral density scores for your hip. If the scores are low in your hip, there is a good chance you may have also lost bone mineral density in your spine.

Tests to Measure Bone Mineral Density

Test	Benefits	Limitations	Concerns
Dual-energy x-ray absorptiometry (DEXA)	• Currently the best predictor of hip fracture • Can measure as little as 2% bone mineral loss per year • Uses 2 different beams to estimate bone mineral density at key sites • Good predictor of fracture at all sites • Low dose of radiation • Widely available • Covered by insurance • Measures bone mineral density of hip, lower spine (L1-L4) and thigh • Accurate • Non-intrusive • Requires little time (less than 10 min.)	• Can't take calcium tablets for 24 hours before test • Can't wear metal in jewelry or clothing during test • May not give accurate results if spinal degeneration has occurred	• Some radiation exposure • Doesn't distinguish between trabecular bone and cortical bone • Does not show changes in bone geometry
Radiographic absorptiometry (RA)	• Uses standard x-ray equipment which is widely available • Low dose of radiation • Non-intrusive	• Requires special equipment and software to analyze results • Measures bone mineral density in finger which does not yet correlate to other sites	• Peripheral sites are typically highest in BMD due to more use and impact • Doesn't show density of either hip or spine • Some radiation exposure
Single energy x-ray absorptiometry (SXA)	• Measures bone mineral density in forearm or heel • Equipment is portable • Low cost	• Part being tested must be submerged in water • Can't take calcium tablets for 24 hours before test • Takes a long time to complete	• Doesn't show density of hip or spine — only measures density of sites tested • Peripheral sites are typically highest in BMD due to more use and impact • Not as accurate as other tests • Some radiation exposure

Test	Benefits	Limitations	Concerns
Peripheral dual–energy x–ray absorptiometry (PDXA)	• Measures peripheral sites such as wrist, heel, or finger • Requires little time • Very low dose of radiation • Equipment is portable • High resolution • High degree of accuracy at sites tested • Quick results	• Expensive	• Doesn't show density of hip or spine — only measures density of sites tested • Peripheral sites are typically highest in BMD due to more use and impact • Not accurate enough to assess effectiveness of osteoporosis medications • Some radiation exposure
Peripheral quantitative computed tomography (pQCT)	• Very accurate • Used in research • Only test that measures both cortical and trabecular bone in the forearm	• Requires CAT scan with special software • Expensive • Test takes a long time	• Delivers high dose of radiation • Often overestimates amount of bone lost
Quantitative ultrasonography (QUS)	• Measures flexibility and total bone strength • No radiation — uses sound waves • Tests peripheral site, usually the heel, wrist, or finger • Not intrusive • Requires little time • Readily available	• Soft tissue and bone type influence readings making results less accurate	• Not as accurate as other tests • Not a good predictor of osteoporosis (if low, other tests are still required) • Doesn't show density of hip or spine — only measures density of sites tested • Peripheral sites are typically highest in BMD due to more use and impact in daily life

HOW TO

UNDERSTAND YOUR BONE MINERAL DENSITY REPORT

The main purpose of obtaining a bone mineral density test is to determine your risk of fracturing a bone. To some degree, your bone mineral density correlates with your risk of fracture. When you receive your scores, you will see a variety of numbers that can be used to help predict your risk. Some of these numbers are actually comparisons to other people's score results.

T-SCORE

The most commonly used score is the T-score. Although it is usually presented as your score, it is actually a statistical comparison of your bone mineral density to others of the same sex and ethnicity. The manufacturer of the densitometry machine includes an expected normal value for this reference population in the software, and your bone mineral density is compared to that number. The expected normal value is called the young adult mean, or young adult average, which is the average peak bone mineral density for people in an age range somewhere between 20 and 40 of the same sex and ethnicity. Unfortunately, not all manufacturers of bone densitometers use the same database. Some cutoff their young adult mean scores at age 29, others at age 40, and most don't differentiate between athletes and non-athletes. As a result of this non-standardization, the significance of your T-scores may vary if you have follow-up tests done on a different machine. Your scores will also mean something different than the T-scores of your friends and relatives.

Your T-score is not your actual bone mineral density (BMD). Your actual bone mineral density value shows up on your test results as grams per area (g/cm^2). Your T-score is the difference between your bone mineral density value and the young adult average. This difference is called a standard deviation (SD). Your T-score tells you how far your bone mineral density is above

> *The lower your T-score, the lower your bone mineral density is in comparison to the average bone mineral density of young adults between 20 and 40 years old with your same ethnicity and gender.*
>
> - *T-score = 0 (your BMD is exactly the same as the average)*
> - *T-score < 0 (shown as a negative number, your BMD is below the average)*
> - *T-score > 0 (shown as a positive number, your BMD is above the average)*

or below the young adult average. So if your T-score equals +1, your bone mineral density (in grams per area) is one standard deviation above the average young adult population for your sex and ethnicity.

> *The formula used to determine your T-score is:*
>
> **(your BMD – average BMD) ÷ the SD of young adult average**

What does this mean to you? Because the main purpose of strong bones is to prevent fractures, consider it in terms of your risk of fracture. For every standard deviation your bone mineral density falls below the average, it is estimated that your risk of fracture doubles. So, if your T-score is –1, you run twice the risk of fracturing that bone as a person with a T-score of 0 (T-score of 0 = a normal risk of fracture and is given a value of 1. This number doubled: 1 x 2 = 2). The doubling occurs cumulatively for each standard deviation. So if your T-score is –2, your fracture risk increases to 4 times greater and if your T-score is –3 the risk is 8 times greater than the normal risk.

> *T-score = 0 (average)*
> *Fracture risk factor = 1*
> *T-score = –1*
> *Fracture risk factor = 2*
> *T-score = –2*
> *Fracture risk factor = 4*
> *T-score = –3*
> *Fracture risk factor = 8*

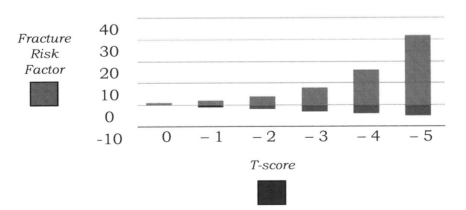

As T-score gets lower, fracture risk increases exponentially

If your doctor tells you your risk of fracture based on your T-score, remember that this is an educated guess. There is really no definitive way to predict your actual risk of fracture. Think of it as you would a standard height/weight chart used by insurance companies. To obtain the data in those charts, researchers measure the height and weight of a certain number of healthy people in a specified age bracket. Then they take the average of those numbers and, based on your comparison to that average, predict your chances of getting a disease such as diabetes or cardiovascular disease.

Researchers can do this because there is a known correlation between obesity and certain diseases. These numbers help researchers understand the relationships that are involved. But height/weight charts are not designed to be predictive databases. They do not consider your percentage of body fat, build, family history, or any other known risk factors. They only focus on one data point — your height and weight on a given day. That number has no magic predictive powers; it is simply a way to compare your height and weight to others in your age bracket. If you weigh 20 pounds above the average, you are not guaranteed a future heart attack. Maybe you've always weighed 20 pounds more than the average person in your age group. A better indicator of how you are doing is to compare your actual height and weight today with your healthy height and weight in your mid-20s. Obviously, this will vary from person to person, as does individual bone mineral density.

In the early 1990's osteoporosis was redefined. It used to mean, "an elderly person with a fragility fracture." Now it is considered a "risk factor for a fracture." Around that same time parameters were set for the risk of fracture and consequently a diagnosis of osteoporosis. Originally T-scores were established as an operational definition of osteoporosis for research and comparison purposes. They were not intended to be references for determining treatment although they have become the standard reference for it.

To repeat: T-scores were developed by researchers as a way to compare bone mineral densities. They were not originally intended to be predictive databases but have evolved into such. What we must remember is that every

Classification of T-score Values Based on the World Health Organization's Evaluation:

- *Normal bone mineral density: T-score ≥ –1*
- *Osteopenia: T-score = –1 to –2.5*
- *Osteoporosis: T-score ≤ –2.5*
- *Severe or advanced osteoporosis: T-score ≤ –2.5 and you have had one or more fragility fractures*

body is unique by design. We are not all built from the same mold, so use these results as they were meant to be used — as comparisons. They can be good estimates but are not the final word.

> *If you multiply your T-score times 10, you can estimate the percentage of bone mineral density you have above or below the norm. A T-score of 1 indicates a 10% greater bone mineral density than the average young adult in your gender and ethnicity. A T-score of –2.5 indicates a 25% lower bone mineral density than the average young adult.*
>
> *If you've had two subsequent bone scans you can compare the results to see how much bone you've lost or gained. For example, if your first T-score was a –1 and your second was a –2.5, your score lowered by 1.5 so you've lost approximately 15% of your bone in the time between your tests.*

Z-SCORE

The Z-score is another number that researchers came up with to understand and explain osteoporosis. It is also a statistical comparison to your bone mineral density. It is similar to a T-score, but adds age, height, and weight to the comparison. By comparing you to others with your same age, build, gender, and ethnicity, you can better understand how you are doing in relationship to your peers. This isn't as good at predicting your bone strength but it can help classify the type of osteoporosis you have, if you have it. Primary osteoporosis is age-related so you will probably have a higher Z-score if yours is primary. Secondary osteoporosis is suspected if your Z-score is lower than –1.5. This type of osteoporosis is caused by some other illness or condition that induces bone loss such as thyroid or parathyroid issues, poor digestion, alcoholism, smoking, or the use of certain medications.

If your Z-score is lower than –1.5, your doctor may order additional tests, including blood or urine tests, to find out if there is an underlying cause of your osteoporosis. This is important to know because treating the underlying condition may be necessary to correct the low bone mineral density.

> *Remember, everyone is different and started out with their own unique peak bone mineral density. A Z-score compares your current bone mineral density to people of your same sex, ethnicity and age as well as your similar height and weight. It's kind of like comparing lemons with limes. They are shaped alike and are both citrus fruits but they aren't the same.*

BONE MINERAL DENSITY (BMD)

A T-score compares your current bone mineral density to people of your same sex and ethnicity, whose bones have just finished growing and are at their peak. A Z-score compares your current bone mineral density to people of your same age, height, weight, gender, and ethnicity. These scores were originally developed as research tools, not as diagnostic scores. The best indicator of your bone density is your actual bone mineral density (BMD).

Your BMD is the amount of bone minerals per square centimeter in the section of bone that was tested on you. Shown as a number followed by g/cm^2, it is your score with no comparisons to anyone else. If your test was done between the ages of 20 and 40, before you went through menopause or any form of major drug treatment, it is a good measure of your peak bone mineral density.

Save these results no matter what age you were when the test was done. Once you have this number, you can compare any future results to it and you will know exactly how much bone you have lost or gained. If you've only had one test, you have no basis for comparison and you cannot tell if you've actually lost any bone.

> ## BMD Is Like Your Bones' Blood Pressure Score
>
> *Think of your BMD scores as you would a blood pressure score. Although there are guidelines established through research, your score is specific to you. For example, the recommended values for blood pressure are 120/80. This is an average healthy score. My blood pressure consistently measures around 112/70 – a bit below the recommended value of 120/80. When I have my blood pressure measured, I don't compare my results to the healthy average for the population, I compare them to my known healthy numbers. If it goes up significantly from my norm, I'll want to evaluate my lifestyle to make sure I'm giving my heart and circulation the best possible environment.*

A Downside of Bone Mineral Density Tests

Bone mineral density scans provide information that helps us estimate the strength of bones, but there is no direct evidence that screening with these tests prevents or reduces fractures. If we become solely dependent on this one predictor, there is a risk of misdiagnosis and overmedication. Although decreasing bone mineral density is a sign that your bone remodeling cycle is out of balance, taken out of context and used by itself, it is not an accurate predictor of fracture. Low bone mineral density is simply one indicator of low bone strength as are loss of height and kyphosis.

Keep in mind that genetics determine your skeletal design, which also plays a role in bone strength. Depending on your genetic makeup, your bones may have a different shape or structure than another person of your same age, sex, and race. If your femur responds to mechanical loading by becoming more structurally efficient but not thicker, it may show up as a borderline or osteoporotic bone because your bone mineral density at that location is lower than in people with thicker bones. This doesn't mean you have osteoporosis. Structurally efficient bones are not weaker bones. They simply use the bone tissue in a more efficient manner, requiring less material for the same strength. Studies performed on mice have shown that this greater structural efficiency is a result of a better response to mechanical loading. When a force is applied to these bones, they react more quickly and effectively than thicker, denser bones. This principle is covered in depth in Chapter 7, the exercise chapter.

Based on everything I've studied and on my experience teaching my BONES Lifestyle classes and workshops, my main concern about relying too heavily on bone mineral density tests is that if the results are low, you may experience unnecessary and excessive anxiety or fear about fracturing a bone. In Chapter 4, I discussed the B for Balance of the BONES Lifestyle. Remember that a

> *If you follow the BONES Lifestyle, you will develop the strength and balance to move with confidence.*

fear of falling leads to overly cautious movement, which causes many falls. Falls are a major cause of bone fracture due to osteoporosis. Many people contact me after their first bone mineral density scan with questions and concerns about osteoporosis. What's amazing to me is that as I talk to them, they are all struggling with an intense fear of moving wrong or falling and breaking a bone. Even strong, healthy people feel fragile after a diagnosis of a below average T-score.

Remember, bone mineral density tests have limitations in their ability to provide consistently accurate results. Your results will vary from one type of test to another as well as from one machine to another of the same type. As with any predictive test, the results are not 100% accurate — they simply provide an estimate of your bone's density at the time of the test. Bone mineral density scans can be skewed by equipment failure, technician mistakes, your build, the thickness of the tissue that surrounds the bone, calcium supplements taken within the past 24 hours, patient movement during the test, or degenerative joint disease, among other things.

One study done in 1991 demonstrated that bone mineral density scans are not necessarily the best predictor of potential fracture. This study showed that low bone mineral density measurements identified only 6% of the women who actually suffered from fractures. This and other research provide evidence that instead of just focusing on BMD scan results to identify at-risk individuals, we should take into account all of a person's risk factors and focus on living a bone-healthy lifestyle such as the one described in this book. Everyone should focus on prevention, not just those identified as "at risk." Balance practice, nutrition, and exercise are the most effective tools available to prevent or manage lifestyle-related osteoporosis.

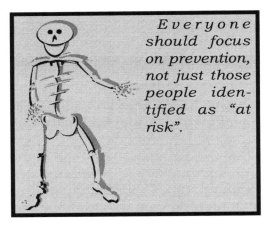

> *Everyone should focus on prevention, not just those people identified as "at risk".*

HOW TO
KNOW WHEN YOU NEED AN OSTEOPOROSIS TEST

Research has shown that bone mineral density tests are a useful tool for identifying people at risk of fracture due to osteoporosis. But, to date, these studies have not provided sufficient evidence to support general screening of all people for osteoporosis. Therefore doctors are not automatically prescribing these tests.

People with multiple risk factors run a higher risk of developing osteoporosis in the future. If this is your situation, or if you are worried about it, then ask your doctor for a bone scan. It's a good idea to get your first bone mineral density scan before menopause, in your 30's or 40's, to determine your peak bone mineral density. Later, when you repeat the test, you will have something to compare your results to. Remember, you cannot determine if you have lost bone with just one test! You can only compare your results with those of other women. Once you've gotten a baseline BMD, the National Osteoporosis Foundation recommends a test at about age 65, unless you present additional risk factors or sustain a fragility fracture.

1ST BONE SCAN

If you are a woman with multiple risk factors, try to get this done before you enter menopause. It is valuable to establish your baseline BMD. Get a full copy of your test results and ask your doctor to review the results with you. Be sure to find out the actual numbers of your bone mineral density in grams per area for each site that was measured. This baseline number is good to have so you can monitor how your bones are changing over time.

Although the T-score can be helpful to see where you fall as compared to the norm of people in your gender and ethnic group, the best determinate of your bone health is to compare subsequent tests to your actual peak bone mineral density. If you can get a bone scan before menopause to determine your personal peak bone mineral density, then you can monitor your own bone mineral density instead of comparing your measurement to a norm. Keep in mind however that bone mineral scan reports are not exactly comparable if you didn't get the scan done on the same type of machine, preferably the exact same machine.

If you have already gone through menopause, then start where you are today. When you receive your test results, look at your scores with your doctor to determine if you may be at a greater risk of fracture. No matter how old you are, use this test result as a baseline. The T-score is a predictor of low bone mineral density, but don't panic if it is low. You may have started with a lower peak bone mineral density than the average person in your category, or your bones may be configured in such a way as to maximize bone strength with less mineral density.

If you have been diagnosed with cancer (especially estrogen-dependant cancer), plan to get a bone mineral density scan before treatment to determine your baseline bone mineral density. Repeat a scan after your treatment ends to see if you have lost any bone during treatment so you can begin a bone therapy program if necessary.

Make sure you save a copy of these results so you can compare them to later test results.

2ND BONE SCAN

Bone growth is a slow process and the most common bone mineral density tests can't measure the small changes that occur over a short time period. Two years appears to be the minimum time period for changes to show up on a bone scan.

If you are at risk, wait at least two years before you ask your doctor to prescribe a second bone scan. If you aren't at risk, you can wait until age 65. Compare your actual bone mineral density value of this scan to your actual bone mineral density value of the previous scan. Has it gone down? If so, now is the time to take more action. Make sure you are following a bone-healthy diet like the one in Chapter 6, doing your weight-bearing resistance exercises like those in the BONES Lifestyle Exercise Program© outlined in Chapter 7, and taking vitamin/mineral supplements as suggested in Chapter 8. Talk to your doctor about medication or other therapy that may be necessary. He may want to run some additional tests to be sure you don't have an underlying disease that is causing the osteoporosis. If you are on medication that depletes bone mineral, you may need to consider other options, such as a different medication.

If the second test indicates the same or higher bone mineral density, stay on track with your BONES Lifestyle and ask your doctor to repeat the test about every three to five years. If the second test shows bone mineral loss, ask for laboratory (blood and urine) tests to determine potential contributing factors, review your lifestyle for ways you can improve your bone health, initiate a course of treatment with your doctor, and continue getting biannual tests for a few years to determine how fast you are losing bone and if your treatment regimen is working. Once your tests indicate a stabilization of bone remodeling, get additional scans every 2 to 5 years, depending on your doctor's recommendation. If at all possible, you should repeat each bone scan on the same instrument and with the same technician. Because this is usually a difficult order, keep in mind that there may be variations in the results from one test to the next due to human or instrument inconsistencies. Just because your bone scan shows a lower than average bone mineral density doesn't mean you will walk out the door and fracture your hip. Use your test results to motivate you toward a healthier lifestyle.

Even if your bone mineral density has decreased, there is still no reason to panic. Osteoporosis is treatable with lifestyle changes and appropriate medications. Work with your doctor to determine the best course of action for you. You may need medication now, or you may be able to take a more conservative approach. No matter what you decide to do, be proactive about your health and be happy that you have discovered this deficiency before a fracture occurs.

IF YOU HAVE ALREADY EXPERIENCED A FRAGILITY FRACTURE

Get a bone mineral density scan to determine your current BMD. A fragility fracture is the only sure sign that you have osteoporosis. This type of osteoporosis is categorized as severe (or advanced) osteoporosis because once you have experienced one fragility fracture you are at a high risk for another. Your doctor will probably order some additional laboratory tests, including blood and urine tests, to establish baseline conditions and to rule out any secondary causes of low bone mineral density. Take the same steps as you would above but follow the Modified BONES Lifestyle Exercise Program for Severe Osteoporosis© shown in Chapter 7. You will probably need to take medication to help build bone mineral density and prevent future fractures. In this case, the best therapy generally includes a combination of medication, supplements, proper nutrition, and exercise. It is very important to incorporate balance exercises into your routine if you have severe osteoporosis to help you prevent falls.

6

Nutrition

Nutrition is known to play an important role in the growth of strong bones and the prevention of osteoporosis. But as you've learned in earlier chapters, no two people are alike. This applies to food choices as well. The foods you eat interact with your genetic makeup and lifestyle to help determine your osteoporosis risk factors. Personal, geographical, economic, social, and cultural factors all influence our diets. You may eat a diet similar to that of other people, but your body will respond to the foods differently. Your taste buds respond to foods in a unique way as well. You have your own preferences and dislikes that influence your food choices.

Nutrient intake directly affects both the development and maintenance of your bones' strength. Your bones need the same nutrients as the rest of your body.

Cross-cultural studies have uncovered a multitude of dietary patterns around the world, and there is no clear connection to one "magic pill" nutrient that will prevent or cure osteoporosis. Interestingly, most people in the United States believe that calcium, (milk in particular) makes strong bones. But cultures such as China, Cambodia, and Ghana rarely consume milk, yet they have the lowest incidences of osteoporosis.

Food Groups

The United States Department of Agriculture (USDA) was created in 1862 to "ensure a sufficient and reliable food supply" and to keep the public informed on subjects related to agriculture. In 1917, the USDA established the first food groups by organizing foods into five different groups based on known nutrient content. These five groups included fruits and vegetables, protein-rich foods (including meat and milk), starchy foods (including breads and cereals), sweet foods, and fatty foods. This concept of food groups became the standard for all future nutrition advice. The groups have changed a bit over the years, but the idea of balancing your diet by getting varied nutrients from different types of foods has remained a successful model.

During the 1950's, the USDA specified the size of a serving and the number of servings the average healthy person should eat per day. This Daily Food Guide included four food groups – milk, meat, vegetable/fruit, and bread/cereal. The thought was that people needed help making wise food choices to meet the recommended daily allowance for necessary nutrients. In 1992, after much debate and numerous attempts at a graphical illustration of a food guide, the Food Guide Pyramid was released. This design made sense and was easily understood: Eat less of the foods towards the top and more of the ones near the bottom.

The idea of a food pyramid caught on and now you can find a food pyramid guide for almost any diet — Asian, Mediterranean, and Vegetarian, among them. I like the idea of the food pyramid because it provides a quick and easy reference for food choices. So I have developed one for a bone-healthy diet based on current research.

The BONES Food Pyramid©

The BONES Food Pyramid includes the variety of foods that will help meet your bone's nutritional needs. I've divided the pyramid into 11 levels based on the bone-healthy nutrients found in the food groups. Try to eat foods from each food group during the week. As you can see, that will include daily servings of vegetables and whole grains.

If you are wondering why I didn't list exact serving sizes or amounts in the **BONES** Food Pyramid, it was intentional. I believe that when we become too focused on the numbers, it's easy to lose sight of the big picture. The food pyramid is a tool to help you evaluate and establish patterns in your eating plan.

Now let's take a look at the research behind the **BONES** Food Pyramid, so you will understand why it is organized this way.

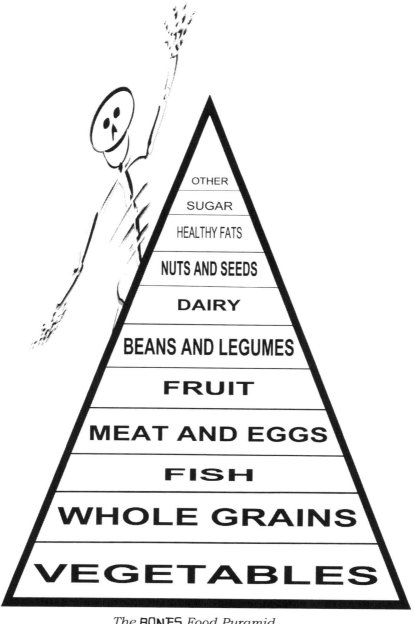

The **BONES** Food Pyramid

The Low-Down on Calcium

Bone has nutrient requirements similar to those of the rest of your body even though many sources claim that "combined with decreases of estrogen during menopause, low calcium intake is the main cause of osteoporosis." As nice as it would be to have such a clear origin, osteoporosis is just not that straightforward.

In one study, premenopausal and postmenopausal women who increased their calcium intake to greater than 1,000 milligrams for at least 18 months significantly reduced cortical and trabecular bone loss in the femoral neck and reduced the incidence of hip fractures. But this is not a permanent improvement. While short-range studies like this have demonstrated lower levels of bone loss with high calcium diets, long-range and cross-cultural studies have been unable to identify a lower risk of hip fracture when people consume a diet high in calcium or milk.

Many cultures eat less calcium than we do in the United States, but have lower incidences of osteoporosis. For example, calcium intake in Japan is lower than in the United States, but the rate of hip fracture in the United States is twice that of Japan. Also interesting is that these high-calcium diets don't seem to have the same positive effects on lumbar vertebrae.

Until recently, most of the studies that had to do with nutrition and osteoporosis involved calcium. From these studies, we have learned some important facts about how our bodies use this mineral. These studies have shown that calcium intake encourages osteoblast (bone building) activity, especially in the limbs. They have demonstrated that the body stores calcium in bone and strives to maintain a positive calcium balance in the blood at all times, borrowing from the storage supply if this balance is disrupted. Since only 1% of your body's calcium is circulating in your blood, 99% is stored in your bones. An average adult body contains about 750 to 1,200 grams of calcium. One percent of that equals 7.5

> On average, an adult female skeleton will reach a peak of about 750 grams of stored calcium.
>
> A middle-aged woman can lose between 0% and 3% of her bone mineral content, which includes calcium, per year. This amounts to a loss of up to 2.25 grams of calcium per year. If this rate of loss continues for 20 years, she will have lost a total of 45 grams of bone mineral.
>
> Osteopenia is a loss of 10% to 25% of your peak bone mineral density, or 7.5 to 18.75 grams of calcium if your peak was at the average 750 grams. A loss of more than 25% of your peak bone mineral density is classified as osteoporosis.

to 12 grams, which is used for normal heart and brain function, blood pressure, metabolism, muscle contraction, nerve transmission, and blood clotting. This circulating calcium also helps you maintain a strong immune system, keeps your brain alert, and reduces fatigue. That one percent even helps keep your vision sharp!

Given the small amount of available calcium that is essential for life, we lose an alarming amount each day — an average of 160 to 320 milligrams (mg). That is approximately 1.2% to 3.8% of our body's available supply lost through metabolism, sweat, urine, and feces, as well as shed skin, nails, and hair. If you do not replace this calcium, your body will take measures to maintain the life-sustaining 7.5 to 12 grams.

An elaborate banking system that balances dietary and stored calcium monitors the blood's supply. If the lost calcium is not replaced by absorption of new calcium from food or supplements, your body will excrete a parathyroid hormone that increases bone resorption (the breakdown of bone). This releases more calcium from the bone's storage supply into the blood, and the life-supporting balance is restored.

As you learned in Chapter 1, problems can arise when the balance of minerals in your bones is depleted for essential bodily functions but is not replaced. If calcium is borrowed from the skeleton and not replaced over the years, the debt can easily compound, leading to significantly lower bone mineral density and osteoporosis. You cannot live with a chronically negative calcium balance without affecting the mineral content of your bones. Fortunately, you can keep the bank from tapping your savings by absorbing as much of this valuable mineral as possible. What is just recently becoming clear is that this is also true for the other essential minerals that are stored in bone including phosphorus, magnesium, and sodium.

As all this information surfaced about calcium, the medical community began to encourage patients to increase their calcium intake and moms began asking, "Did you drink your milk

> *To figure out the number of milligrams of calcium in a serving of food, read the label and multiply the percentage of calcium by the number 10. That number is the amount of calcium in milligrams. For example, if the label says 35% calcium % daily value, multiply 35 by 10 and your serving contains 350mg of calcium.*

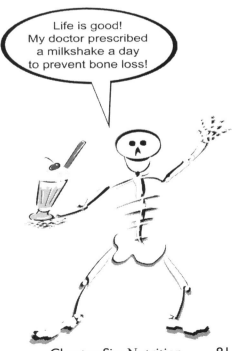

Life is good! My doctor prescribed a milkshake a day to prevent bone loss!

today?" But cases of osteoporosis continue to increase even as people consume more calcium in response to their doctor's (and mother's) recommendations. While there is sufficient evidence to show that adequate calcium is important in the battle against osteoporosis, the healthiest amount has not yet been established.

Most of the studies that have been done to determine calcium retention in bones are short-term studies. This means that they only measure the effectiveness of calcium intake over a short period of time. The few longer-term studies seem to suggest that the body adapts to calcium intake over an extended period of time, and high intake doesn't necessarily reduce a person's risk for osteoporosis. In one study, people who drank 8 ounces or less of milk per week didn't face a greater risk of fracture than people who drank 16 or more ounces of milk per week.

So what does all this mean?!?

> *Estimates are that up to 35% of Americans are deficient in calcium. The average daily intake for adult women is below 500mg. That's less than one-half the recommended amount of 1000 to 1500 mg.*

Your Bones Depend On At Least 22 Different Nutrients

Clearly, calcium is a necessary nutrient for bone health, but it is also clear that it is not the magic pill that will prevent or cure osteoporosis. New research indicates that at least 22 different nutrients affect bone density. The effects of an imbalance of these nutrients are seen in the results of scientific studies, including:

1. If the ratios of phosphorus to calcium or protein to calcium are not balanced, calcium absorption appears to decrease.

2. A link has been found between adequate vitamin D consumption and 37% fewer hip fractures.

3. A link was found between high intakes of fruit during childhood and high femoral neck bone mineral density in adult women. The same link was not evident in women who had a high consumption of milk products or vegetables during childhood.

4. Low levels of vitamin B12 have been linked to low bone mineral density in men's hips and women's spines. High daily doses of B12 (1500mcg) and folic acid, also known as B9 (5mg), reduced hip fractures by 80% in stroke patients.

5. A deficiency of copper or vitamin B6 in the diet may weaken the collagen matrix in bone and lead to lower bending strength and greater brittleness.

6. In one study a combination of vitamin D and calcium showed a reduction in fracture rate for people older than 60 by about 30%.

The Vitamin D Connection

A deficiency in vitamin D is more common than previously recognized. This can have a significant influence on the development of osteoporosis. Vitamin D is necessary for the absorption of calcium and for bone resorption (the activity of the bone crushers). But as with all nutrients in our diet, there is no evidence that vitamin D alone prevents osteoporotic fractures. It works in combination with other vitamins and minerals to maintain healthy bones.

Our bodies convert sunlight into vitamin D. In general, you need about 10 minutes of sun exposure a day to absorb an adequate amount of vitamin D. If you are house-bound, office-bound, or live in a place where the sun rarely shines, be sure to consume foods that are rich in vitamin D or consider taking vitamin D supplements. Oily fish like salmon, mackerel, sardines, and herring contain this vitamin, as do eggs, liver, and cod liver oil. Because it is an important vitamin that is hard to get in the diet, many foods are fortified with vitamin D, including milk and breakfast cereals.

Magnesium and Potassium: The Forgotten Minerals

A magnesium or potassium deficiency can affect the calcium balance and a deficiency of either may also contribute to osteoporosis. Fur-

A study done at Oregon State University looked at the relationship between calcium and protein and bone mineral density in women during their first 3 years of menopause. Their results suggest that consuming adequate amounts of calcium and protein at this age does not significantly slow bone loss over a 12-month period.

However, other studies have shown benefits from increasing calcium intake in premenopausal women and women who were 6 years or more postmenopausal. This discrepancy may be due in part to the fact that the majority of bone loss occurs in the first years after menopause begins. Calcium and protein intake may not be able to overcome this natural decline.

ther research is needed in order to understand the benefits of these minerals, but studies have shown that magnesium is an extremely important mineral in skeletal metabolism.

About 1% of the mineral in bone is magnesium. This mineral influences the turnover of calcium and the metabolism of the collagen matrix. If the magnesium content of bone mineral decreases, the mineral crystals grow larger and become more brittle, a common occurrence found in the bones of osteoporotic women. These changes make bone more susceptible to fracture. One study found that eating foods high in dietary magnesium (grains, fish, and vegetables) was associated with increased bone mineral density at the hip for both men and women. However, because these foods also tend to be high in potassium and other valuable nutrients, the specific effects of magnesium were not clearly identified.

High dietary potassium intake also has a positive relationship to bone mineral density in adults. Potassium has been shown to decrease urinary calcium excretion and bone resorption (the breakdown of bone) while increasing bone formation. Foods rich in potassium help buffer acids in the body and maintain a normal pH so your body doesn't need to borrow calcium from the bones to neutralize acids. Fruits and vegetables contain significant amounts of potassium but unfortunately this mineral tends to be deficient in many American diets.

> *Bone mineral density is positively affected by intake of fruits and vegetables, which are packed with potassium. This valuable mineral slows the excretion of calcium.*

What Are You Eating?

You don't eat nutrients, you eat food that contains nutrients, and no single nutrient or food group can build strong bones on its own. Research has shown that at least 22 key nutrients work together to build strong, healthy bones. These include: calcium, magnesium, phosphorus, potassium, boron, copper, manganese, silica, sulfur, zinc, vitamin A, vitamin B5, vitamin B6, vitamin B9, vitamin B12, vitamin C, vitamin D, vitamin E, vitamin K, protein, essential fatty acids, and fiber.

The following chart in the "How To" section gives examples of foods containing the bone-healthy nutrients. For each nutrient, the food groups are listed in order of importance. The food groups that are listed first provide the greatest amounts of the nutrient.

HOW TO

FIND FOODS CONTAINING BONE-HEALTHY NUTRIENTS

ESSENTIAL MINERALS (required in relatively large amounts)	FOUND IN THESE FOODS (in order of quantity of nutrient)
CALCIUM *Important mineral that provides bone strength* *Deficiency is common*	• **Dairy** (yogurt, cheese, milk, buttermilk) • **Vegetables** (artichokes, broccoli, bok choy, okra, parsnips, peas, squash, sweet potatoes, collard greens, spinach, turnip greens, mustard greens, beet greens, dandelion greens, Chinese cabbage, kale) • **Seafood** (sardines, salmon, perch, crab, clams, trout, cod, haddock, tuna) • **Beans** (tofu, soybeans, black, white, chick peas, kidney, lentils, lima, navy, pinto, cowpeas) • **Fruits** (figs, kiwi, raspberries, oranges, bananas, papaya) • **Nuts and Seeds** (almonds, sesame) • **Other** (blackstrap molasses, fortified cereals and flours)
MAGNESIUM *Assists with calcium uptake and the metabolism of the collagen matrix* *Deficiency is common*	• **Grains** (buckwheat, bran cereal, quinoa, bulgur, oat bran, brown rice, wheat germ, corn meal, oatmeal, amaranth, millet, corn) • **Fish** (halibut, pollock, tuna, haddock, shrimp) • **Vegetables** (beet greens, spinach, artichokes, broccoli, parsnips, swiss chard, peas, pumpkin, okra, spinach, summer squash, sweet potatoes, potatoes, tomato paste, kelp) • **Beans** (navy, great northern, lima, black, white, soybeans, cowpeas, tofu, lentils, chick peas, black-eyed peas) • **Nuts and Seeds** (brazil, almonds, pine, cashews, peanuts, hazelnuts, pumpkin, sesame, squash) • **Fruits** (bananas, apples, figs, prunes, plantains, plums, grapefruit) • **Dairy** (yogurt) • **Other** (blackstrap molasses, chocolate, coffee)

PHOSPHORUS

Important mineral providing bone strength

Intake is usually adequate or overconsumed

- **Grains** (barley, buckwheat, oat bran, rice, wheat, bran, bulgur, flour, corn)
- **Fish** (cod, crab, flounder, haddock, lobster, mussels, oysters, prawns, salmon, sardines, scallops, tuna, mollusks, pollock, swordfish)
- **Dairy** (cheese, dry milk, milk, yogurt)
- **Meats** (eggs, bacon, beef, chicken, duck, ham, lamb, pork, sausage, turkey)
- **Beans** (soybeans, lentils, great northern, navy, lima)
- **Nuts and Seeds** (sesame, almonds, brazil, cashews, peanuts, pistachios, walnuts, coconut, hazelnuts, macadamia)
- **Vegetables** (spinach, peas, parsley, mushrooms, potatoes)
- **Fruit** (dried fruits)
- **Other** (chocolate, yeast)

POTASSIUM

Neutralizes metabolic acids to preserve calcium, slows excretion of calcium, and increases bone formation

Deficiency is common

- **Vegetables** (tomatoes, sweet potatoes, yams, potatoes, winter squash, beet greens, collard greens, spinach, carrots, broccoli, peas, brussels sprouts, artichokes, cabbage, parsnips, pumpkin, kohlrabi, mushrooms, rutabagas, beets)
- **Fruits** (dates, raisins, bananas, prunes, plantains, peaches, apricots, apples, cantaloupe, honeydew melon, oranges, grapefruit, watermelon, avocados, plums, papayas)
- **Beans** (white, lima, lentil, kidney, soybeans, split peas, cowpeas)
- **Fish** (clams, halibut, rockfish, cod, tuna, trout, haddock)
- **Grains** (buckwheat, bulgur, barley, oat bran, whole wheat)
- **Meats** (duck, pork, beef, chicken, turkey)
- **Nuts and Seeds** (chestnuts, sunflower)
- **Dairy** (yogurt, milk, buttermilk)
- **Other** (blackstrap molasses, cocoa)

TRACE MINERALS *(required in smaller amounts)*	FOUND IN THESE FOODS *(in order of quantity of nutrient)*

BORON

Aids in calcium absorption

No established RDA

- **Nuts and Seeds** (almonds, brazil, cashews, hazelnuts, peanuts, walnuts)
- **Fruits** (raisins, prunes, apples, apricots, avocados, bananas, dates, grapes, oranges, peaches, pears)
- **Beans** (kidney, chick peas, lentils)
- **Vegetables** (turnip greens, beet greens, broccoli, carrots, celery, olives, onions, potatoes)
- **Other** (honey)

COPPER

Aids in bone formation and helps build a strong collagen matrix

Deficiency is common

- **Fish** (oysters, lobster, crab, clam, mollusks)
- **Meats** (veal, beef, goose, duck, lamb, liver)
- **Grains** (barley, buckwheat, rice, bulgur, whole wheat, couscous, oat bran)
- **Vegetables** (seaweed, tomatoes, grape leaves, mushrooms, radicchio, turnip greens, beet greens, collard greens, asparagus, swiss chard, potatoes, cabbage, sweet potatoes, spinach, artichokes)
- **Beans** (soybeans, white, tofu, chickpeas, lentils, cowpeas, lima, great northern, kidney)
- **Nuts and Seeds** (chestnuts, sunflower, cashews, brazil, walnuts, hazelnuts, tahini, pumpkin, pistachios, pine, coconut)
- **Fruit** (dates, plums)
- **Other** (coffee, salt, tea, tap water, chocolate)

MANGANESE

Aids in the formation of bones and connective tissue

Intake tends to be low

- **Grains** (oat bran, bulgur, barley, buckwheat, rice, wheat bran, wheat germ, rice bran, whole wheat, oats, rye, couscous)
- **Fruits** (pineapple, blueberries, loganberries, blackberries, raspberries)
- **Vegetables** (peas, green beans, yellow beans, lemon grass, spinach, okra, seaweed, grape leaves, endive, turnip greens, beet greens, collard greens, carrots, broccoli, potatoes, cabbage, sweet potatoes)
- **Nuts and Seeds** (pine, coconut, hazelnuts, soy, pecans, chestnuts)
- **Beans** (chick peas, lima, soybeans, white, cowpeas, lentils, navy, tofu, great northern)
- **Fish** (mollusks)
- **Other** (tea, salt, spices, coffee, chocolate)

SILICA

Aids in calcium absorption

No established RDA

- **Grains** (barley, oats, rice)
- **Vegetables** (lettuce, parsnips, asparagus, onion, cabbage, cucumber, leek, celery, rhubarb, cauliflower and swiss chard)
- **Fruit** (strawberries)
- **Nuts and Seeds** (sunflower)

SULFUR

Essential for collagen formation

No established RDA, intake is usually sufficient

- **Meats** (eggs, beef)
- **Beans** (pinto, kidney, lima, lentils, navy, white, chick peas)
- **Vegetables** (garlic, onion, spinach, jicama, alfalfa sprouts, broccoli, asparagus, cabbage, mustard greens, watercress, parsley, swiss chard, sweet potatoes, tomatoes, brussels sprouts, turnips, seaweed)
- **Nuts and Seeds** (sunflower, cashews, walnuts, almonds, sesame, coconut)
- **Grains** (corn, oats, wheat germ)
- **Fruits** (avocados, watermelon, raspberries)
- **Dairy** (cheese, milk)
- **Other** (drinking water, chocolate, carob, coffee, tea, turmeric)

ZINC

Assists with calcium uptake and immune function

Deficiency is common

- **Fish** (oyster, crab, lobster, clam, swordfish)
- **Meats** (chicken, lamb, turkey, beef, duck, pork, liver)
- **Beans** (lentils, black-eyed peas, soybeans, white, chick peas, pinto, lima, kidney)
- **Grains** (barley, buckwheat, whole wheat, wheat germ, bulgur, cornmeal, rice, couscous)
- **Nuts and Seeds** (sunflower, cashews, tahini, pumpkin, pine, coconut, cashews)
- **Vegetables** (peas, mushrooms, tomatoes)
- **Dairy** (milk, cheese, yogurt)
- **Other** (fortified cereals)

VITAMINS	FOUND IN THESE FOODS
(required in varying amounts)	*(in order of quantity of nutrient)*

VITAMIN A (BETA CAROTENE OR RETINOL)

Strong anti-oxidant retards aging process

Intake tends to be low

- **Vegetables** (pumpkin, sweet potatoes, carrots, spinach, winter squash, red sweet pepper, bok choy, dandelion greens, beet greens, collard greens, turnip greens, mustard greens, dandelion greens, Chinese cabbage, kale, lettuce, tomatoes, broccoli, peas, asparagus, endives, onions, parsley)
- **Meats** (turkey, beef, chicken, liver, giblets, eggs)
- **Fruits** (cantaloupe, mangoes, apricots, papaya, plums, tangerines, plantains, cherries, watermelon, peaches)
- **Beans** (soybeans, cowpeas)
- **Dairy** (cheese, milk, yogurt)
- **Fish** (pickled herring, clams, mackerel, tuna, bluefish)
- **Other** (fortified cereals, cod liver oil)

VITAMIN B5 (PANTOTHENIC ACID)

Antioxidant that stimulates the healing process

Deficiency is common

- **Meats** (beef, chicken, turkey, pork, goose, duck, lamb, eggs, liver, veal)
- **Grains** (couscous, brown rice, bulgur, corn, oat bran, whole grains, buckwheat)
- **Vegetables** (mushrooms, leafy greens, endive, watercress, cauliflower, tomatoes, brussels sprouts, cucumber, broccoli, summer squash, arugula, zucchini, peas, sprouts, seaweed, radishes, potatoes, sweet potatoes)
- **Dairy** (yogurt, milk)
- **Fish** (rockfish, trout, whale, lobster, salmon, catfish, halibut)
- **Beans** (cowpeas, kidney, mung, soybeans, navy, lentils, split peas, lima)
- **Fruits** (avocados, blueberries, blackberries, grapefruit, oranges)
- **Nuts and Seeds** (sunflower, chestnuts)
- **Other** (fortified cereals, coffee, tea)

VITAMIN B6

Helps build a strong collagen matrix

Deficiency is common

- **Fish** (tuna, cod, halibut, haddock, swordfish, rockfish, salmon, trout)
- **Meats** (beef, turkey, duck, chicken, pork, eggs, ham, liver)
- **Vegetables** (potatoes, tomatoes, broccoli, sweet potatoes, brussels sprouts, spinach, sweet red peppers, sweet green peppers, okra, sauerkraut, onions, turnip greens, kohlrabi)
- **Grains** (rice, buckwheat, oatmeal, wheat germ, cornmeal, barley, bulgur, wheat flour)
- **Fruits** (bananas, prunes, plums, plantains, avocados, oranges, grapefruits, grapes, mangos, raisins, pineapples)
- **Beans** (lentils, soybeans, lima, navy)
- **Nuts and Seeds** (pistachios, chestnuts, peanuts, sunflower, coconut)
- **Other** (fortified cereals)

VITAMIN B9 (FOLIC ACID)

Helps break down homocysteine levels (high homocysteine levels raise risk of osteoporosis fracture)

Intake tends to be low

- **Grains** (brown rice, cornmeal, wheat flour, white rice, corn, wheat germ, buckwheat)
- **Beans** (lentils, pintos, chick peas, black, navy, cowpeas, kidney, soybeans, great northern, white, lima)
- **Vegetables** (okra, spinach, asparagus, collard greens, turnip greens, broccoli, mustard greens, brussels sprouts, artichokes, lettuce, beets, peas, sweet potatoes, parsnips, cabbage, endives)
- **Meats** (beef, liver, eggs)
- **Fruits** (papayas, citrus, bananas, raspberries)
- **Nuts and Seeds** (chestnuts, sunflower)
- **Other** (fortified cereals, baker's yeast)

Vitamin B12

Important for normal growth and immune function. Deficiency can cause balance problems

Intake tends to be low

- **Fish** (oysters, clams, crab, salmon, sardine, cod, trout, herring, pollack, flounder, lobster, halibut, swordfish, rockfish, catfish, shrimp, haddock, tuna)
- **Meats** (beef, turkey, lamb, pork, chicken, eggs, liver, organ meats)
- **Dairy** (cheese, yogurt, milk)
- **Other** (fortified cereals)

Vitamin C

Strong antioxidant, important for collagen and connective tissue formation

Intake tends to be low

- **Fruits** (oranges, grapefruit, peaches, papaya, guava, kiwi, limes, lemons, strawberries, cantaloupe, cherries, pineapple, mango, tangerines, raspberries, plantains, starfruit, blackberries, honeydew melons)
- **Vegetables** (red sweet pepper, green sweet pepper, brussels sprouts, bok choy, kohlrabi, broccoli, peas, sweet potatoes, tomatoes, cauliflower, kale, collard greens, asparagus, red cabbage, turnip greens, mustard greens, sauerkraut, rutabagas, okra, potatoes)
- **Nuts and Seeds** (chestnuts)

Vitamin D

Assists with calcium uptake and absorption

Deficiency is common

- ** Exposure to sunlight is the best source but be cautious of overexposure
- **Fish** (salmon, mackerel, sardines, herring)
- **Meats** (eggs, liver)
- **Other** (cod liver oil, fortified milk, fortified cereals)

Vitamin E

Strong antioxidant retards aging process, enhances bone quality

Deficiency is common

- **Vegetables** (tomatoes, spinach, turnip greens, dandelion greens, carrots, beet greens, pumpkin, sweet potatoes, broccoli, sweet red peppers, asparagus, collard greens, mustard greens, parsnips, kale)
- **Nuts and Seeds** (sunflower, almonds, hazelnuts, pine, peanuts, brazil)
- **Fruit** (mangos, papayas, raspberries, blackberries, peaches, apricots, oranges, blueberries, kiwi, nectarines)
- **Fish** (crab, sardines, orange roughy, herring, rockfish, salmon)
- **Beans** (soy, pinto, kidney, lima)
- **Meat** (duck, chicken)
- **Other** (olive oil, peanut oil, corn oil)

VITAMIN K

Positively affects bone metabolism by reducing bone breakdown

Intake tends to be low

- **Vegetables** (kale, collard greens, turnip greens, beet greens, spinach, mustard greens, broccoli, brussels sprouts, onions, asparagus, carrots, endive, lettuce, parsley, cabbage, peas, cauliflower, kale, sauerkraut, okra, pumpkin, celery, cucumber, tomatoes, green beans, yellow beans, sweet green peppers)
- **Fruits** (prunes, blackberries, blueberries, kiwi, plums, grapes, pears)
- **Beans** (soybeans and other soy foods, mung, cashews, chick peas, lentils)
- **Fish** (tuna)
- **Spices** (cilantro, thyme)

ESSENTIAL NUTRIENTS	FOUND IN THESE FOODS
	(in order of quantity of nutrient)

PROTEIN

Necessary structural component of bone, part of the collagen matrix that gives bone flexibility

Often overconsumed

- **Meats** (duck, chicken, turkey, eggs, beef, pork, veal, lamb)
- **Fish** (halibut, salmon, tuna, haddock, rockfish, salmon, cod, trout, crab, shrimp, swordfish, flounder, clams, sardines, shrimp, lobster, scallops)
- **Dairy** (cheese, milk, soy milk, yogurt)
- **Beans** (soybeans, tofu, white, chick peas, lentils, kidney, black, pinto, navy, great northern, lima, cowpeas)
- **Nuts and Seeds** (peanuts, pumpkin, sunflower, flax, almonds, walnuts, pine, cashews)
- **Grains** (couscous, bulgur, oat bran, buckwheat, quinoa, corn, wheat germ, oats, rice, whole grains)
- **Vegetables** (broccoli, spinach, potatoes)

ESSENTIAL FATTY ACIDS

Enhance calcium absorption and increase bone protein synthesis

Deficiency is common

- **Fish** (salmon, mackerel, sardines, anchovies, tuna)
- **Nuts and Seeds** (flax, walnuts, pumpkin, brazil, sesame, pine, pistachios, sunflower, almonds, peanuts, cashews, hazelnuts, macadamia)
- **Fruits** (avocados)
- **Vegetables** (kale, spinach, purslane, mustard greens, collard greens, olives)
- **Meats** (eggs, chicken)
- **Other** (flaxseed oil, olive oil)

> *Research repeatedly shows a positive link between fruit and vegetable consumption and healthy bones. Numerous studies have shown that women who consume the most plant-based foods are the least likely to get osteoporosis.*

Looking at this chart, it becomes clear that strong bones require a team effort by many different vitamins, minerals, and nutrients. Research has shown that most people in the United States are deficient in a majority of the necessary bone-building nutrients. Part of the reason for this is the typical American diet — filled with ready-made, processed foods. When you look at the assortment of foods that provide the essential nutrients for strong bones, it becomes apparent that a diet packed with a variety of nature's provisions is the most beneficial for your bones. The best way to obtain all the bone-healthy nutrients and to get them working as a winning team is by eating a balanced diet filled with fresh vegetables, fruits, whole grains, beans, nuts and seeds, fish, lean meats, and dairy — the basis of any healthy diet.

I find it significant that plant-based foods are a source of most of the bone-healthy nutrients. Vegetables contain all of the nutrients that are necessary for bone health except for vitamins D and B12. Fruits provide all the necessary nutrients except protein, zinc, vitamin B12, and vitamin D. Whole grains, beans, nuts, and seeds are also good sources for most of the bone healthy nutrients.

Many of the countries in Asia, Africa, and the Mediterranean that have low incidences of osteoporosis consume diets that are traditionally plant-based — high in vitamins, minerals, fiber, and phytochemicals. In contrast, these foods are typically underconsumed in the United States — where osteoporosis is prevalent. So instead of asking yourself if you drank your milk today, a more important question might be, "Did you eating your veggies and fruits today?"

> *It will be years before science uncovers the interactions between all the elements of nourishment and their effects on bone health.*

Eat Your Colors

In 400 BC Hippocrates said, "Let food be your medicine and medicine be your food." The nutrients we consume through the food we eat help us grow, give us energy, and assist our body's normal functions. But there is much more to a healthy diet than just proteins, carbohydrates, vitamins, and minerals.

Phytochemicals are the compounds that give plant foods their color, flavor, and scent. The definition of phytochemical actually includes all compounds in a plant, including nutrients. But they are not usually classified as nutrients in the same sense as carbohydrates, fats, proteins, minerals, and vitamins.

> *The most naturally colorful foods contain the greatest number of healthful compounds, including vitamins, minerals and phytochemicals. When selecting fruits and vegetables, choose the deepest reds and purples, the darkest greens and the brightest yellows and oranges.*

Instead, the word phytochemical is generally used to describe all the other substances that make up the plant. Phytochemicals do not generate energy or build cells, but they do play an essential role in health. They serve as antioxidants, anti-inflammatories, immune system stimulants, antibacterials, antivirals, and they provide natural detoxification. But probably of greatest interest for people dealing with osteoporosis is the ability of phytochemicals to regulate hormone metabolism.

Phytochemicals are the substances that give plants their color, flavor, and scent. Therefore, it would follow that plants with the most vivid colors, flavors, or scents are filled with active phytochemicals. Remember when your mom or grandma told you to eat something of each color?

> *Scientists have identified many phytochemicals, but are nowhere close to identifying them all or understanding how they work together with nutrients to prevent disease and create good health.*

> The following foods contain phytochemicals that boost bone mineral density and remodeling and may help prevent or manage osteoporosis:
>
> - *Onions*
> - *Parsley*
> - *Bananas*
> - *Soybeans*
> - *Tea (black or green, not herbal tea)*
> - *Tomatoes*
> - *Prunes (in studies done on animals, prunes actually reversed bone loss)*

They were on to something. Not only are colorful foods fun to eat, but the colorful foods you eat are the best disease-fighters. Studies have shown that phytochemicals play a role in preventing cancer, heart disease, diabetes, osteoporosis, stroke, cataracts, and urinary tract infections. The protective properties of phytochemicals are many and, as with vitamins and minerals, the best way to get them is through the foods you eat.

John Suave, executive director of the Wild Blueberry Association of North America said it well. "It may be that the goal of five fruits and vegetables a day is really about color. You can paint the image of health, but you need all the colors to do that — red, green, orange, and blue — some of each every day."

Colorful foods are rich in a variety of vitamins, minerals, and phytochemicals that act together to build strong bones. We know that bone metabolism requires coordination between the bone crushers (osteoclasts) and the bone builders (osteoblasts). Combinations of nutrients can positively influence this process, particularly by inhibiting the osteoclasts that break down old bone.

pHinding Your Food on the pH scale

Other current research is focusing on the effects of an acidic or alkaline blood pH on osteoporosis. The pH scale ranges from 0 to 14. A pH of 7.0 is neutral. A pH below 7.0 is acidic and a pH above 7.0 is alkaline. Human blood should be slightly alkaline with a pH of 7.35 to 7.45. If your pH drops below or rises above this range, you risk disease.

The concern for people at risk of osteoporosis is an overly acidic pH in the body, a condition called **metabolic acidosis**. If the blood becomes acidic, your body will attempt to neutralize it by drawing alkaline minerals such as calcium, magnesium, potassium, sodium, and zinc into the blood. As you learned in Chapter 1, if your diet doesn't contain enough minerals, your body will borrow from its storage facility in the bones by increasing the osteoclasts (bone crushers) activity and decreasing the osteoblasts (bone builders) activity. But if your body is chronically acidic, even if you are getting the necessary nutrients in your diet, you will not be able to maintain their storage supplies.

The chart in the following "How To" section shows some of the foods that are acid-forming and some that are alkaline-forming.

An acidic pH can be caused by a diet high in acid-forming foods, emotional stress, a toxic environment, or an immune response. The typical American diet is high in acid-forming foods such as meats, fish, cheese, and fats. It is low in alkaline-forming foods such as fruits and vegetables. While some protein in the diet is necessary for bone flexibility, it's not uncommon for Americans to ingest twice the necessary amount, which can lead to chronic low-grade metabolic acidosis and loss of bone mineral. Fruits and vegetables, on the other hand, help buffer acids in the body, which appears to help preserve mineral content in bone.

It's important to balance your diet with foods of all types, including some acid-forming foods and some alkaline-forming foods, keeping in mind that you want to maintain a slightly alkaline pH in your blood.

Osteoporosis is rare in cultures that have predominantly alkaline forming diets such as those of the Chinese, Africans, and Mayan Indians.

Vitamin and Mineral Robbers

It is important to include the necessary nutrients in your diet, but your body won't be able to use these nutrients if you are not absorbing them. It is unclear why some people easily absorb nutrients while others do not. But it is clear that a number of factors can decrease the absorption of nutrients from food including autoimmune diseases, gastrointestinal problems, ingestion of certain medications, excesses of other nutrients, and age, among others.

There are many thieves looking to steal the nutrients that you take in. These thieves prevent your body from properly absorbing vitamins and

HOW TO

FIND ACID AND ALKALINE FORMING FOODS

ACID FORMING

VEGETABLES
- carrots
- peas
- potatoes

FRUITS
- cranberries
- plums
- pomegranates
- prunes

NUTS AND SEEDS
- brazil nuts
- cashews
- hazelnuts
- peanuts
- pecans
- walnuts

BEANS AND LEGUMES
- black beans
- chick peas
- green peas
- kidney beans
- lima beans
- pinto beans
- red beans
- soy beans
- white beans

DAIRY
- butter
- cottage cheese
- cow cheese
- cow milk
- goat cheese
- processed cheeses
- rice milk
- sheep cheese
- soy milk

GRAINS
- amaranth
- barley
- buckwheat
- corn
- oat bran
- rice
- rye
- spelt
- wheat
- wheat germ

ALKALINE FORMING

VEGETABLES
- asparagus
- beets
- broccoli
- brussel sprouts
- cabbage
- cauliflower
- celery
- cucumbers
- daikon
- eggplants
- garlic
- grasses(barley and wheat)
- leafy greens
- mushrooms
- onions
- parsley
- parsnips
- peppers
- pumpkin
- rutabaga
- sauerkraut
- seaweed
- spirulina
- sprouts
- squash
- tomatoes
- watercress

FRUITS
- apples
- apricots
- avocados
- bananas
- berries
- cantaloupe
- cherries
- currants
- dates
- figs
- grapefruit
- grapes
- honeydew melon
- lemons
- limes
- mangos
- nectarines
- oranges
- papayas
- peaches
- pears
- pineapple
- tangerines
- watermelon

NUTS AND SEEDS
- almonds
- chestnuts
- flax seeds
- pumpkin seeds
- sprouted seeds
- squash seeds
- sunflower seeds

ACID FORMING

FISH
- carp
- clams
- lobster
- mussels
- oyster
- salmon
- scallops
- shrimp
- tuna

MEATS
- beef
- lamb
- pork
- rabbit
- turkey
- venison

FATS
- canola oil
- corn oil
- lard
- safflower oil
- sesame oil
- sunflower oil

ALKALINE FORMING

BEANS AND LEGUMES
- lentils

DAIRY
- almond milk
- yogurt

GRAINS
- millet
- oats
- quinoa
- wild rice

FISH
- none

MEATS
- eggs

FATS
- cod liver oil
- flax oil
- olive oil

OTHER ACID FORMING PRODUCTS
- aspartame
- beer
- chemical additives
- coffee
- colas
- distilled vinegar
- drugs(medical and recreational)
- hard liquor
- herbicides
- pesticides
- wine

OTHER ALKALINE FORMING PRODUCTS
- apple cider vinegar
- baking soda
- bee pollen
- fruit juices
- green juices
- green tea
- herbal teas
- mineral water
- molasses
- most herbs
- organic milk
- probiotic cultures
- sea salt
- spices(cinnamon, curry, ginger, mustard, chili)
- tempeh
- tofu(fermented)
- veggie juices
- whey protein

minerals, and they interfere with good health. Some diseases that rob calcium and other nutrients, such as rheumatoid arthritis and juvenile diabetes, cannot be prevented, nor can liver disease or malabsorption diseases. But you may be unknowingly ingesting nutrient robbers and sabotaging your body's balance.

There are some bandits that should be eliminated from the lives of anyone interested in bone health. Tobacco is a major culprit, accounting for roughly one in eight hip fractures. The risks are lower in former smokers, so if you smoke, quit smoking as soon as possible to slow the rate of your bone loss. Likewise, heavy alcohol use has been associated with a greater incidence of both hip and vertebral fractures.

While tobacco and alcohol are easily identified, some of the nutrient robbers act more like sneaky cat burglars. Phosphorus is an essential mineral for bone health, but too much of it may actually decrease the amount of calcium in your body. Phosphorus binds to calcium, so these two minerals need to be evenly matched in your diet or excess phosphorus will look for calcium to bind with, removing it from bone if necessary. Some researchers are concerned that diets high in phosphorus, including excess protein or soft drinks, can rob your bones of necessary calcium. But according to the Linus Pauling Institute at Oregon State University, "a controlled study of young women found no adverse effects of a phosphorus-rich diet (3,000 mg/day) on bone-related hormones and biochemical markers of bone resorption when dietary calcium intakes were maintained at almost 2,000 mg/day." At this time, researchers see no convincing evidence to demonstrate that a high intake of dietary phosphorus adversely affects bone mineral density. However, the fact that many people consume phosphate-containing soft drinks and snack foods in place of milk and other calcium-rich foods does cause concern, as this lack of calcium in the diet could be considered a risk for poor bone health.

People typically absorb between 10% and 60% of the calcium they ingest. If you ingest 300mg of calcium (the amount available in 1 cup of milk) and absorb 60% of it, you will absorb 180mg of calcium. But if you only absorb 10% of the calcium, you will have only added 30mg to your body's available supply. The difficulty comes in knowing the amount of nutrients your body actually absorbs. At this time there is no way to measure the amount of a nutrient you actually absorb.

The verdict is still out, but excess caffeine intake may also rob calcium from your bones. If you drink the equivalent of more than four 8–ounce cups of brewed coffee per day, you may be upsetting your bone's mineral balance. It's a good idea to limit your caffeine to less than 540 mg per day. Most soft drinks contain somewhere between 40 and 60 mg of caffeine per 12–ounce serving while 8 ounces of tea contains between 40 and 60 mg. Depending on how it's brewed, 8 ounces of coffee may contain anywhere between 80 and 175 mg. Remember, certain medicines such as Anacin and Excedrine also contain caffeine (between 32 and 65 mg) so if you take these, be sure to consider it as part of your daily total.

Protein and high quality essential fats are important for healthy bones, but too much of either can disrupt your bone's remodeling cycle. Furthermore, hydrogenated vegetable oils have been found to decrease the absorption of necessary nutrients such as vitamin K. For overall good health, 50 to 60 grams of protein per day and less than 50 grams of fat are good numbers to shoot for. Salt depletes calcium and other vital minerals in bone so try to keep your salt intake below 2,000 mg/day. One teaspoonful of salt contains about 2,000 mg of sodium.

A lot of the foods we eat contain nutrient robbers although researchers have yet to determine how detrimental these foods are. It is not nec-

> *A study done at Penn State indicated that high amounts of saturated fat from meats and dairy can weaken bones. Men under 50 who ate the most saturated fat had about 4% less bone density than the other men in the study.*

> *For strong bones, try to limit vitamin and mineral robbers in your food choices. Some commonly used nutrient robbers include:*
>
> - *sodium (salt)*
> - *caffeine*
> - *saturated fats*
> - *hydrogenated vegetable oils*
> - *colas*
> - *processed foods*
> - *sugar*
> - *alcohol*

essary, and probably not even possible, to completely eliminate all of the mineral robbers from your diet, but it is important to be aware of them because the impact of all the potential bone robbers adds up.

Diet Equals The Sum of All Foods

Good nutrition must be a lifetime habit. If you stop eating a balanced, bone-healthy diet, you will lose the benefits that you gained. Your body depends on consistently solid nutrition to maintain good health and strong bones. In many cases, the results of different studies contradict each other or are inconclusive. But one thing is certain — there is a clear connection between nutrition and bone health. Nutrition is one of the most important elements of a BONES Lifestyle and as scientists continue to study bone health, a deeper understanding of all these interactions will help further identify the best ways to manage and prevent osteoporosis.

HOW TO

SELECT A BALANCE OF BONE-HEALTHY FOODS

The **BONES** Food Pyramid is a handy tool designed to help you monitor your bone-healthy nutrient intake. Here is a simple way to utilize the pyramid.

When my children were ages 5 and 3, I made a traditional food pyramid out of a piece of cardboard cut into a triangle. I covered the cardboard with felt and drew the food groups on with a sharpie marker. Each child chose a color and I cut out little felt squares of felt in their colors. They enthusiastically placed a marker for the foods they ate on the correct food group. I found it a helpful tool to monitor my own daily intake as well and had almost as much fun recording my meals as they did. Each day we would try to fill in all the levels with our colored markers to make a perfect triangle. Over time, we no longer needed the felt board pyramid to maintain balance in our diets and even now at the ages of 19 and 17, I still hear my kids say things like, "I need to eat another fruit today" or "I need something with some protein in it."

You don't need to make a felt board of the **BONES** Food Pyramid. Instead, make four photocopies of the pyramid on the next page. You will use one copy per week. Each time you eat something, record your food selections with a mark in the appropriate level. At the end of each week, your pyramid should be shaded evenly. Fill out a pyramid each week for a total one month.

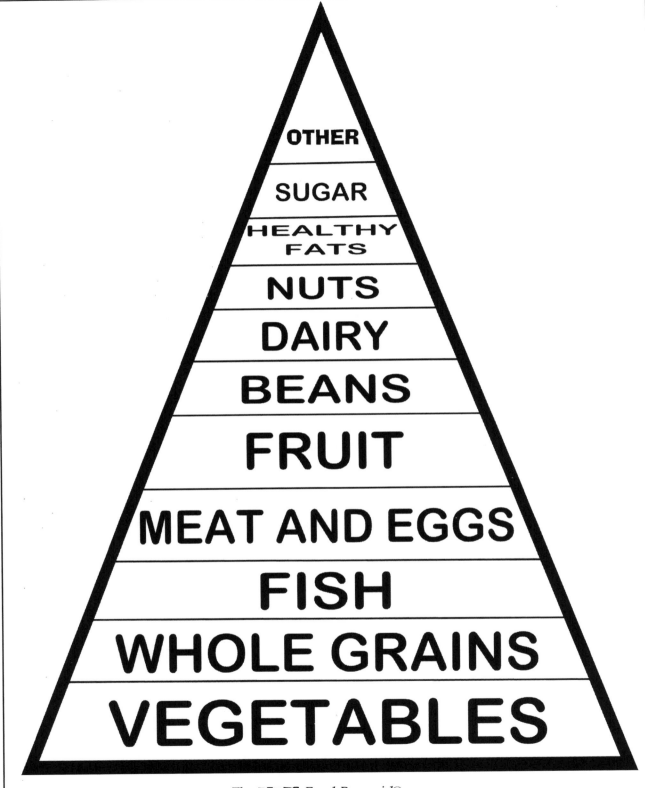

The BONES Food Pyramid©

7

Exercise

In previous chapters, you've learned that osteoporosis is not simply a matter of calcium deficiency. A healthy lifestyle filled with nutritional food and regular exercise is essential for strong bones. In fact, research has shown that exercise is probably our most valuable tool for the prevention and treatment of osteoporosis.

Some studies show an increase in bone density when sufficient calcium intake is combined with an active lifestyle. Other studies indicate that exercise combined with medication provide the greatest protection against osteoporotic fractures. But a consistent finding throughout research is that exercise is an essential component of any bone-health program. It decreases stress, and increases the production of estrogen, which slows down the activity of the bone-crushers

> *Study after study has confirmed that daily weight-bearing exercise is the best way to maintain and improve bone strength at any age.*

> *Both men and women can suffer less age-related bone loss if they exercise in ways that challenge the skeleton. Physical activity increases bone mineral density even in your 70s and 80s.*

> *Animals that were challenged with weight–bearing resistance exercises demonstrated dramatic improvements in bone strength, and it took more energy to fracture the bones of these animals. Interestingly, this added strength came with only a moderate increase of about 5% bone mineral density. The new bone was added to the areas of the bones that had the greatest stress, while areas of low stress didn't increase in bone density.*
>
> *Other studies done on adult rats have also shown that exercise increases the amount of collagen (the foundation that holds the bones together).*

called osteoclasts and increases the work of the bone builders called osteoblasts. Exercise also increases nerve stimulation and blood flow to the bones. This encourages nutrient flow to the bone cells, builds the protein collagen content and stimulates the osteoblasts so they work harder forming new bone.

Exercise improves muscle strength, coordination, and balance, all of which reduce the risk of fracture even without the benefits of increased bone strength. Another condition that is closely related to osteoporosis is the age-related decrease of skeletal muscle called sarcopenia. As you age, you can lose up to $\frac{1}{3}$ of your muscle mass, due in part to inactivity. When muscle mass decreases, your muscles don't perform as well. Consequently, they don't challenge your bones to the same degree and they don't provide the necessary support for your skeletal system. This can lead to frailty, weakened bones, difficulty balancing, poor posture, and a greater risk of falling.

Fortunately, there are movements that increase the strength and flexibility of bones and, at the same time, improve muscle strength, coordination, and balance. The best exercises for building both bones and balance are weight-bearing resistance exercises.

Remember from Chapter 1 that the remodeling system is responsible for breaking down and building up old bone. The system monitors the loads being placed on bone. When a load is applied to a bone through impact, weight-bearing activity, gravitational pull, or mechanical force, it creates strain on the bone, which signals the remodeling system to kick into action.

Some research suggests that these signals are in the form of electrical impulses triggered by the nervous system. The remodeling system responds to these signals, and if the actual strain is greater than the anticipated strain, bone is added to the surface where the greatest strain occurs. If the actual strain is lower than anticipated in an area, bone will eventually be removed from that area. Thus, the bone gets stronger in sections where it is most needed without adding additional weight. With this understanding, you can see how important it is to load all of your bones through full-range, three-dimensional movements to provide strength and functionality to the entire skeletal system.

During childhood, new bone is formed at a faster rate than old bone is destroyed so bones change shape and grow bigger and stronger. Regular weight-bearing exercise during this period of growth can significantly improve bone mass and structure and lead to long-term skeletal health. Although the bone mineral density decreases somewhat if the activity is stopped, the changes to bone shape and size seem to be maintained. This is good news because bone shape and size are more important to bone strength than are measurable changes in bone mineral density.

You say you didn't lead an especially active childhood? Don't fear. While it's a bit more difficult to transform adult bones, they still respond to mechanical stress with changes to size, shape, density and increased strength. Adult bones just require a greater load and/or a load that lasts longer.

Athletes practice specific movement patterns over and over again until they develop muscle memory. Then their body easily repeats the movement when needed. The **BONES** Lifestyle Exercise Program teaches movement patterns that strengthen the muscles and bones around the locations most often affected by osteoporosis.

When you first learn a new exercise, you must concentrate on which muscles to contract so you can move freely and balance at the same time. To train the voluntary muscles to engage correctly on command, focus on the muscles that must contract during the exercise and monitor your form in a mirror. Try each movement using a wall or table for assistance. When you do it right, with good balance and no pain, pause and make a mental list, noting how each part of your body feels (feet, legs, abdominals, back, etc.). Then, as you continue to practice the exercise, remind yourself

Exercise during childhood and your teenage years builds bone density, while exercise during adulthood maintains or rebuilds bone density.

Studies done on postmenopausal women who exercise for strong bones show that when they stop exercising, they lose the bone density they had gained. However benefits gained from exercise during childhood cause the bones to adapt in ways that are longer-lasting. In one long-term study done at Oregon State University, children who gained bone density through an impact-based exercise program still showed measurable benefits 8 years later.

to repeat that same feeling and try to make each movement identical. In response, your muscles will develop a memory and move smoothly and more powerfully throughout the exercise.

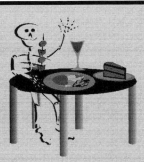

Treat your exercise routine as if it were a fine four-course meal. Begin slowly with the cocktail as a warm-up that will increase blood flow to your muscles, then move into the appetizer and perform smaller versions of the movements you will ask your body to perform in the main dish, where you challenge your muscles with added resistance. After your exhilarating workout meal, cool-down with a relaxing range-of-motion stretch that treats your body with the delight of a decadent chocolate dessert.

Principles of Exercising to Build Strong Bones

To build strong bones, there are some key principles you must be aware of. While getting your heart rate up is beneficial for your heart and lungs, it does little to build stronger bones. Below are the six key principles of building bones.

1. Your bones will adapt to external stress by getting stronger.

2. Only bones that are attached to the muscles being challenged will get stronger.

3. If you stop exercising, your added bone density will decrease.

4. If you've lost more bone or your bones haven't fully developed yet, you have the potential for greater improvement.

5. As you get closer to your goal, the effects of training become smaller.

6. Listen to your body and avoid over-exercising to preserve bone mineral density, maintain postural alignment and prevent fractures.

HOW TO
PREVENT FALLS

Remember in Chapter 4 when I had you practice falling by rolling onto your bed? That exercise is designed to create a muscle memory so that if you are falling and cannot stop the fall, you will land as safely as possible. In this chapter you will learn some exercises to help prevent falls. Here are three of the most important exercises you will learn in this chapter.

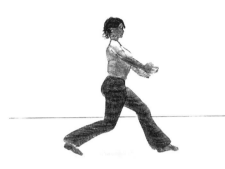

FORWARD LUNGE

If you catch your foot on a carpet or tree root causing you to lose your balance and fall forward, you can prevent a fall by getting your foot out in front of your body to stop your body's forward momentum.

SIDE LUNGE

If you catch your foot on a curb or some other object and begin to fall to the side, you can stop the fall by getting your foot up and over the object and out to the side to stop your momentum.

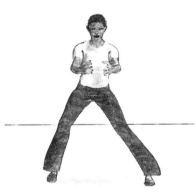

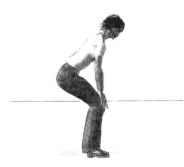

SQUAT

If you slip on ice or lean back too far and start to fall towards the back, you can prevent a fall by bringing your hands to your thighs, bringing your chest forward and pushing your bottom backwards.

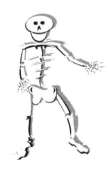

Your bones will adapt to external stress by getting stronger

Your body adapts to its environment. If you don't drink enough water, your body will retain water to keep you hydrated through the dry spell. If you don't eat enough or don't get proper nutrients from your food, your body will conserve energy by storing fat, and your metabolism will change to keep you alive. If you spend an extended period of time sitting, your body will adapt to sitting with a decrease in cardiovascular function, muscle strength, and bone strength. Your goal is to provide the best possible environment to encourage your body to be strong, flexible, and energetic.

Regular exercise is an important part of the "best environment" for your body. Strength training challenges the bones to positively adapt by increasing strain in short powerful bursts followed by a period of rest. The bone cells interpret this stimulus as a safety threat and activate the following protective modifications:

- Increase the density of the outer surface of cortical bone (the chocolate part of the Butterfinger).
- Align trabecular tissue, collagen fibers, and mineral crystals with peak stresses.
- Increase density in bones that experience the most stress and maintain or decrease density in bones that experience the least stress.

There are two primary ways we can stimulate these responses — by increasing force or by adding impact.

Increase Force. First, we can increase the magnitude of the load by increasing the force on the bone. Weight–bearing exercises increase force because gravity is an external force on the body. To stand or walk in gravity requires effort.

But in order to build bone we must increase force beyond our normal activities. A great way to do this is by strengthening the muscles that attach to the bone. As the muscles get stronger, they pull harder on the bone. When we add a weighted

Your body adapts to your lifestyle providing strength where it is needed. If a muscle or bone is overloaded, it will respond by getting stronger. If, on the other hand, a muscle or bone is not being used, the body will put its energy some place it is needed. Inactivity leads to atrophied bones and muscles. An atrophied bone changes little in overall appearance, keeping the same general shape and contour. But the cross-pieces of trabecular tissue and the outer cortical shell become thinner, leaving the bones more porous and fragile.

vest or belt, hand weights, or resistance such as exercise bands, the external force is even greater. Testimony to this is that weight lifters have some of the highest bone density among athletes.

Osteoporosis can affect any bone in your body but because the most common injuries related to osteoporosis occur in the hip, spine, and wrist, the **BONES** Lifestyle Exercise Program focuses on strengthening the muscles that attach to these pivot points. By doing exercises that strengthen the abdominals, back, hips, thighs, buttocks, wrists, and forearms, you will support your bones, move more gracefully, and build bone density in key areas.

The **BONES** Lifestyle Exercises work many muscle groups at the same time to provide greater functional strength and balance training. An additional benefit of these exercises, is that they often eliminate or decrease chronic nagging pain such as back pain.

Add Impact. The second way we can stimulate bone growth is to shock the skeletal system. As stated above, to make bone stronger you must overload it. The amount of force combined with the time to reach peak force makes a difference when developing bones. You can increase both force and time by adding impact. The best impact exercise to develop bone strength is a jump. Jumping achieves peak force quickly and powerfully. The sudden shock surprises the skeleton, and it responds by building itself up to prevent future damage.

Why is this? One theory is that the jolt of landing causes mild electrical impulses from nerve cells that stimulate the bone builders. Force-sensitive plates set into the ground can record the peak-force of a landing. Jumping creates a peak force of 2 to 8 times the person's body weight and the peak force is reached in 0.034 seconds. A single, sudden incident of this amount of force literally "shocks" the system. Weight lifting creates a peak force of 3 to 7 times the body but it takes 3 times longer to reach that force. Consequently, it doesn't create the same shock effect. Running and walking can reach 1 to 3 times body weight but take up to 9 times longer to achieve that peak force.

It is important to jump correctly. Jumping rope, jogging, or bouncing on a mini trampoline don't create the desired response, although all of these activities can be fun. Unfortunately, this type of repetitive loading can actually break down bones if done extensively over time. If you run every day, your bones will initially respond by getting stronger but over time they can develop mechanical fatigue and instead of responding positively to the stimulus of landing on each step, their structure will begin to break down. Long-distance runners, although usually very fit, typically have lower bone density than other athletes and often suffer from a variety of stress fractures in their lower bodies.

If you've ever had a fatigue fracture (also called a stress fracture), you've experienced the effects of mechanical fatigue due to repeated loading. A bone with a fatigue fracture is weakened to the point of developing a small crack. If the osteoclasts and osteoblasts are not given time to clean out and seal the crack, it will grow in the same manner a crack on the windshield of your car grows.

On the other hand, a jump-stop stimulates the skeleton. Take the example of a gymnast dismounting from uneven bars. The force of the landing shocks the skeleton, and because the landings come at varying times, the skeletal system can't predict when the next impact will occur, and it is startled each time. To prevent injury, the skeleton responds by getting stronger to accommodate the force in case it happens again. Studies consistently report strong bones in competitive gymnasts, dancers, high jumpers, basketball players, and other athletes who experience multidirectional, nonsequential landings.

Another benefit of the jump-stop is that it is a safe way to create the feeling of falling. As your body responds to this sensation successfully, the muscles remember, and the brain and body

A fatigue, or stress, fracture is similar to the breakdown of building materials that occurs on older bridges. As each car or truck drives across a bridge, the material in the bridge (metal, concrete, or wood) is loaded and shifted. At the same time the ground around the bridge is moving and changing shape, causing different loads. After thousands of cars and trucks have driven across a bridge, the building material will experience **mechanical fatigue,** *usually in the form of small cracks. If not repaired, these cracks will grow possibly to the point of failure. You don't want to be in the car on the bridge when that happens!*

develop new neural pathways so that when you truly are in danger of falling, your muscles automatically 'catch' you. Many falls are prevented this way.

Only bones that are attached to the muscles being challenged will get stronger

Exercise for building bone is site specific. The bones that are attached to working muscles are the ones that will benefit. But many muscles work together to create movement either as movers or as stabilizers.

For example, if you swing a hammer or play a piano, you engage the muscles in your forearm and hand that attach to the wrist bones. But at the same time, the muscles of your upper arm that are attached to the humerus will contract as stabilizers. All of the bones that are attached to working muscles will benefit. But unless you are contracting muscles around your hip as you move your arm, your hip bones won't get stronger.

Impact from jumping or kicking directly affects the thigh bone and pelvis, thus increasing bone mineral density in the hip. Contraction of the muscles in the thighs, buttocks, and abdomen also increase bone density in the hip because these muscles attach to the hip/pelvic region. Contraction of back, shoulder, and abdominal muscles help build strong bones in the spine. These are also necessary posture muscles so when they are strong, your body's alignment and your balance will improve.

Studies done on athletes show greater muscle strength and bone mineral density in highly trained body parts. Tennis players consistently show a greater bone mineral density in the bones of the dominant arm — the arm that swings the racket to hit the ball. Soccer players show higher leg muscle mass than control groups and markedly increased bone mineral content and bone mineral density at the femoral necks of both legs (top of the thigh bones) and at the lumbar spine region (lower back).

If you stop exercising, your added bone density will decrease

To maintain bone health and fitness levels, you must make exercise a lifetime habit. If you stop exercising, you will eventually lose the benefits you gained. It's important to find ways to include the bone-building exercises in your weekly routine. Studies have shown that it only takes two weeks to lose the benefits muscles gain from a resistance-training program. This will affect the adaptive response of your bones. Additional studies have shown that people who are on prolonged bed rest lose bone rapidly and become osteoporotic within the first 12 weeks of inactivity. At 12 weeks, they reach an equilibrium state, during which less bone is lost but bone turnover is still greater than it would have been if the person was living a normal, active life.

If you've lost more bone or your bones haven't fully developed yet, you have the potential for greater improvement

The initial values of your peak bone mineral density determine where you will end up. You reach your peak bone density around age 25 when your skeletal growth is complete. Mechanical loading during the growing years is essential for a strong, functional skeleton. Many kids run and jump without much prompting, but if you didn't engage in active play, sports, or dance as a child, the peak bone mineral density in your arms and legs may be 30% to 50% lower than average.

After about age 25, your bones stop growing bigger in size, and the effects of exercise shift to preventing bone loss and rebuilding lost bone. The good news is, if you've lost more bone, you have the potential to gain more bone back through exercise, nutrition, and medical therapy. The reverse of this principle can be demonstrated in terms of losing weight. If you start off with an initial weight of 203 pounds and set a goal weight of 145 pounds, you have 58 pounds to lose. If your friend sets the same goal weight but starts off at 178 pounds, she only has to lose 33 pounds. Although you have a higher initial value, you also have the potential to lose more weight than she does and you can see more improvement. So with that in mind, don't be too disheartened if you find out you have lost more bone. That just means you have the potential for greater improvement. There's always a silver lining.

As you get closer to your goal, the effects of training become smaller

When you first begin an exercise program, you are likely to experience big changes, but these changes diminish as you get stronger. As your

> *A sedentary lifestyle leads to bone loss. When patients are placed on total bed rest, bone is lost at an average rate of 4% per month! Adding movement while lying down offers minimal, if any, improvement to bone density and calcium excretion. Adding resistance exercises while in bed slightly improves bone density. But, interestingly, just standing quietly for 2 to 4 hours per day without added exercise appears to reverse the loss in bone mineral that was induced by bed rest.*

bones get stronger, a different or greater load is required to challenge them.

Aerobic exercise programs designed to increase your heart rate challenge the cardiovascular system (heart and lungs) but only minimally challenge the bones. After the first minute or so of the repetitive loading common to aerobic exercise, the cellular response of bones switches off. For example, if you've never walked for exercise, your bones will initially respond to a new walking program by laying down greater density to protect you from injury. But after a while, your bones get comfortable with walking and your skeletal remodeling system gets lazy. If it could talk, your skeleton would say, "Why do I need to change? I know what to expect and I'm strong enough to do this."

Exercise patterns must be different from daily activity and varied enough to get bone to respond and reorganize. You have to surprise the skeletal system with diverse exercises that require unusual loading patterns or quick changes in movements in order to have the greatest effect on bones. The **BONES** Lifestyle Exercise Program works the joints through multidimensional movements that keep the skeleton on its proverbial toes.

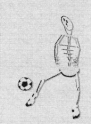

Tennis, softball, dance and soccer are better bone-building sports than running, cycling, or swimming.

But beware if you have advanced osteoporosis. It is not recommended that you participate in high impact sports like these because of the risk of serious injury. If you do have advanced osteoporosis, you can still safely enjoy the benefits of bone-building exercise. It is recommended that people with advanced osteoporosis work with a physical therapist or personal trainer who understands osteoporosis and follow the modified exercise program at the end of this chapter.

Listen to your body and avoid over-exercising to preserve bone mineral density, maintain postural alignment and prevent fractures

Forget the "no pain, no gain" mantra of the 1980s. Contrary to the saying, you do not need to experience pain to strengthen your body. Exercise should be pleasurable. Common mistakes people make when exercising include: trying to do too much too soon, performing exercises that are too advanced, using incorrect form, or doing too many repetitions. The benefits of exercise come over time and are more effective if maintained over time. When you try to do too much, you will wake up hurting the next day and won't want to exercise again anytime soon. Start slow and work

> *We have a saying in our house when we stay up too late and we know we will be sorry when the alarm goes off in the morning. "That's tomorrow guy's problem. Right now tonight guy is having fun!" To date, tomorrow guy has never been happy. Don't put the burden on tomorrow guy by over-doing exercise today.*

> *Many people experience aches and pains as they age. When assessing pain, it helps to consider a pain scale of 1 to 10 with 1 being little or no pain and 10 being extreme pain. In general, if you are experiencing pain that you perceive to be over 3 on the scale, have a doctor check it out. Other clues that indicate pain may require more attention is if your pain is different from pain you've experienced before, is ongoing, limits your daily activities, or keeps you awake at night.*

your way up to more difficult movements. When you are ready for more, your body will tell you. Likewise, if your body needs a gentle workout on some days, it will tell you that too. Listen to your body's signals and respect them.

Over-exercising can actually cause you to lose bone. Female athletes who train so hard that they stop menstruating increase their risk of osteoporosis. This condition, called amenorrhea, is typically a result of malnutrition, low body weight, and inadequate body fat because these women expend more energy than they take in. The imbalance alters hormone production and decreases the amount of estrogen. With less estrogen, the osteoblasts stop building as much new bone tissue and the result is a net loss of bone.

Overworking muscles that are not properly trained can tear the muscle fiber or damage connective tendons and ligaments. This type of injury may alter your gait and affect the way a bone is loaded. A bone that is repeatedly loaded at the wrong angle is more likely to fracture.

Even when the bones are aligned correctly, repetitive loading done over a long period of time can lead to mechanical fatigue and a fatigue (stress) fracture. Fatigue fractures occur without excessive loading but with repetitions of higher than normal loads. This causes the bone structure to break down. If you take on a project that requires repetitive movements such as lifting or shovelling, begin training for a marathon, or dramatically increase your activity level in an exercise program, you may experience a fatigue fracture.

Fatigued bone has less elasticity and strength. If the fatigue continues at a rate that is faster than the repair can occur, the bone will weaken to the point of breaking. It becomes a race between microdamage and microrepair within the bone. Fatigue failure may occur after different amounts of additional stress depending on your genetic makeup and anatomy. But there is evidence that your neuromuscular system has built-in protection to prevent overloading the bone. If you override this protective mechanism with intense emotional reactions such as fear or excitement or because of an extremely competitive drive, your muscles may fatigue sooner. When a muscle fatigues, the strain on the attached bone increases but the neuromuscular system doesn't step in to prevent overloading so the likelihood of a fatigue fracture is greater.

Furthermore, the time it takes a bone to fatigue gets shorter as you age and if you have osteoporosis, fatigue damage is even more likely to occur with overexercise. The message is clear: You must listen to your body! If you feel pain or suspect you may have a stress fracture, take a break from your normal workouts, change your patterns of movement, and give your body a chance to heal. Your bone cells will repair the damage but can do so only at a limited rate.

Fatigue Fractures vs. Fragility Fractures

It is important to clarify and distinguish between fatigue fractures and fragility fractures.

A *fatigue fracture* is the result of repetitive microdamage typically due to excessive mechanical stress on the bone. If the osteoclasts and osteoblasts don't have a chance to repair the microdamage, cracks can appear in the bone and weaken it.

A *fragility fracture* is a fracture caused by decreased bone strength due to osteoporosis and occurs with very little mechanical stress on the bone. It is a measure of true osteoporosis. The bone structure has weakened to the point of failure. If you have experienced a fracture after very little force was applied to a bone, it is likely that you have osteoporosis and you are at risk for additional fragility fractures.

When I first began teaching fitness classes at the age of 23, I took on a rigorous schedule. Although I was very fit at the time, my previous exercise schedule had included training to increase my strength and endurance for soccer and softball. When I got my new job, I enthusiastically jumped into teaching 3 to 5 high impact aerobics classes per day and before long the ball of my right big toe began to hurt whenever I stepped on it. An x-ray didn't show anything but my doctor diagnosed it as a stress fracture and recommended time off. I returned a few weeks later for a second x-ray and the results showed that microdamage had indeed occurred in the bone. This second x-ray showed a line where the fracture and repair had occurred.

As I learned the hard way, a bone that is "fatigued" will hurt but will not show visible signs of damage on an x-ray until after the repair process has begun. Then the changes can be viewed in an x-ray.

AMOUNT OF STRESS ADDED TO BONES	RESULTS
Not enough	Disuse osteoporosis, Greater likelihood of fragility fracture
Normal	Maintain bone mass
Moderate overstrain	Increase bone mass
Severe overstrain	Increase bone mass but risk fatigue fracture

Collapsed Vertebrae

One in ten women over age 65 has a collapsed vertebra due to a compression fracture. Unlike other osteoporotic fractures, vertebral compression fractures don't usually follow a fall. Most spinal fractures that cause a vertebra to collapse occur after straightening the spine from a flexed (forward bending) position — a common movement when lifting a bag of groceries, making a bed, or opening a window. The force is more dangerous if the movement occurs quickly.

Forward flexion of the spine puts extra pressure on the front part of the vertebra and can cause it to collapse into a wedge shape. This is especially true if the flexion includes lifting or lowering an object. Studies have shown that the forces exerted on the spine when lifting about 200 lbs. would crush the vertebra of a relatively inactive senior. Smaller loads may not crush the bone but can certainly cause significant damage. How much do you think that flower pot on your back deck weighs? You know, the one you moved last week so the flowers could get better sun?

The wedge fracture is one type of vertebral fracture. Other types of fractures that can occur to the vertebrae are crush fractures (a collapse of the back or entire vertebral body), biconcave fractures (collapse of the center of a vertebra) or a fracture of one of the transverse or spinous processes.

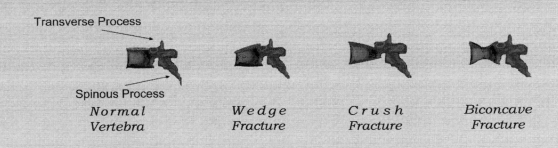

Transverse Process

Spinous Process

Normal Vertebra   *Wedge Fracture*   *Crush Fracture*   *Biconcave Fracture*

Squat To Protect Your Vertebrae

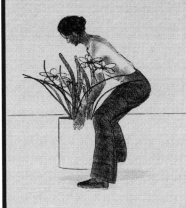

A squat is a safe way to decrease the risk of a fractured vertebra when lifting an object. To squat, keep your torso straight and tilt it on a diagonal as you bend your knees and push your hips back as if you were going to sit down on a chair. Instead of rounding your back forward, squat every time you lift or lower an object.

As you lift, keep the object as close to your body and your center of gravity as possible because for each inch that the load is moved away from your center of gravity, the forces on your spine increase exponentially by a factor of 9. This same principle holds true when lifting free weights as you may choose to do in the exercise program.

Correct lifting

HOW TO

THE BONES LIFESTYLE EXERCISE PROGRAM©

SAFETY PRECAUTIONS

Some motions are known to increase the risk of spinal fracture in people with osteoporosis of the spine. To protect a fragile spine, you will want to avoid exercises that involve rounding your back when bending forward. This is called trunk flexion. When you round your torso forward, most of the movement occurs in the mid to lower back — the mid-thoracic to lumbar region of

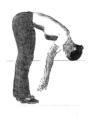

Avoid trunk flexion

the spine. A disproportionate amount of pressure is placed on these vertebrae when the spine is flexed. If your vertebrae are weakened due to osteoporosis, they can collapse. Exercises that may require trunk flexion include sit-ups, straight leg kicks, somersaults, and toe touches.

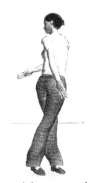

Avoid excessive torso rotation

Excessive torso rotation, or twisting your torso, is also dangerous if you have weakened vertebrae. When you twist your torso, most of the movement occurs in the center section of your spine, around the thoracic vertebrae. Small finger-like projections on each vertebra called transverse processes catch the vertebra above it during rotation. Over-rotating the spine can place too much stress on a weak bone causing a little 'finger' to break off. Some exercises that involve this motion include spinal twist, windmills, and opposite toe touches.

To protect a fragile hip, avoid exercises in which you open your leg too high out to the side. This movement is called hip abduction. Overdoing hip abduction can place extra stress on the upper part of the thigh bone where it

attaches to the pelvis socket — the femoral neck. Some exercises that involve these movements include side leg kicks, splits, and straddle jumps.

Incorrect hip abduction

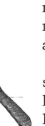

Correct hip abduction

Many movements require you to open your leg out to the side, and it is a safe motion if done correctly. If you move your leg out to the side, you should be able to do so easily while keeping your torso upright and feel no pressure, strain, or pinching in your outer thigh or lower back when you lift your leg. Never swing your leg out to side with force.

Needless to say, in the **BONES** Lifestyle Exercise Program, these movements are not performed. Chapter 10 offers ways to modify your daily activities so you can avoid these movements throughout your day as well.

It is recommended that you do these exercises with someone who can observe and help critique your form so you know you are performing the exercises safely. Don't hesitate to show this book to your physical therapist or personal trainer. They can evaluate your current fitness level and any limitations you have, and help you get started with this program.

FOR NEW EXERCISERS AND PEOPLE WITH SEVERE OSTEOPOROSIS

If you are new to exercise, have fractured a bone, have received multiple bone density scans indicating your bone mineral density is clearly decreasing, or if your doctor identifies additional medical conditions that are causing osteoporosis, then you should do modified exercises. In the section following the regular **BONES** Lifestyle Exercise Program in this chapter, there is a section titled Modified **BONES** Lifestyle Exercise Program For Severe Osteoporosis. Read through the full workout first to be sure you understand the exercises, and always respect your body's signals. If an exercise hurts — don't do it.

READ THE EXERCISE DESCRIPTIONS

Even if you've done one or more of these exercises before, be careful to read the entire description of each exercise, paying careful attention to the alignment cues. To prevent injury, proper form is essential. It is always better to do fewer repetitions with correct form than many repetitions with poor form. In other words, do not repeat poor form.

Some of the exercises may seem easy or too basic to you. Don't be misled. By the time we reach our 30s most of us have developed habitual movement patterns. What we think we are doing and what we are actually doing may be very different. As you practice these movements correctly, you will develop strength and enjoy the rewards of better posture and stronger bones.

Perform each of these exercises 3 times per week. They do not all have to be on the same day. All of the strength training moves should be done without weights until correct form can be repeated easily for three sets of 8 to 12 repetitions. Once you are ready, add either a weighted belt, a close-fitting weighted vest, or hand weights. Begin with 1 to 4 pounds and increase by ½ pound every other week if you are doing the exercises regularly. You will work up to a maximum of 10% of your body weight. If you use a vest or belt, spread the weight evenly around your hips. If you use hand weights, it is important to relax your shoulders and neck. You can either rest the weights on your hips or allow your arms to hang straight down by your sides.

Rules of Engagement

A major focus of the **BONES** Lifestyle Exercise Program is to develop muscular support to protect your spine. You can protect your spine while you are moving by engaging your core abdominal muscles. The core abdominal muscles are deep internal "girdle-like" muscles, sometimes called the pelvic girdle. Although it seems simple enough to say contract your core, this concept is foreign to many people. Many people have never even heard of the "core." You don't need to know the names of all the muscles of the core, nor do you need to individually contract them. Instead, let's use a visualization to help you find your abdominal core. Think of your pelvis as a bowl filled with pancake batter. When your core abdominal muscles are engaged, your bowl will sit flat on the counter. This is called a "neutral pelvis." In this position, your tailbone points down toward the floor and the lower curve of your spine is stable. It's not hard to get your pelvis into a neutral position. All you need to do is pull your belly button in toward your spine as if a string were attached to the back of your belly button and someone was pulling it straight behind you.

But a neutral pelvis alone is not enough to provide full support for your spine. Many people round their shoulders forward and slump when they pull their belly button in, as if they were doing a sit-up, and this is hard on the vertebrae and the vertebral discs. To protect your entire spine, you must engage the upper back muscles with the abdominal core so that the upper curve of your spine is also supported in a neutral position. You can do this by pulling your shoulder blades back and down — as if heavy velvet curtains were hanging off of them. As you engage the upper back muscles in this way, keep your rib cage level — sitting flat on the shelf above your pelvic bowl. In this position, you should feel the muscles under your armpits tighten. This stabilizes your shoulder girdle.

To help you remember this connection, I've come up with what I call my Rules of Engagement. These rules apply to all movements — even simple chores like putting dishes away or unloading clothes from a dryer.

1st Rule of Engagement: The abdominal muscles and upper back muscles work together as a team. Whenever you engage your upper back muscles, you must engage your abdominal muscles by pulling your belly button in toward your spine. This will tilt your pelvis into a neutral position and stabilize your pelvic girdle. The opposite is also true. If you engage your abdominals, you must contract your upper back muscles by rolling your shoulders back and down to bring your rib cage into a neutral position and stabilize the shoulder girdle.

2nd Rule of Engagement: Every time you raise your hands above your shoulders, you are engaging your upper back muscles so you must pull your belly button in toward your spine to tilt your pelvis into a neutral position.

WARM-UP

ROLL-DROP-LOCK

- I've come up with an easy way to maintain the Rules of Engagement and I call it the Roll-Drop-Lock. This exercise will train your muscles to bring your spine into a neutral position so the rib cage and pelvis are both neutral and your spine is stable. I will mention this frequently throughout the exercise program as a reminder to set your rib cage into a neutral position over a neutral pelvis.
- To do the Roll-Drop-Lock, you can sit or stand. Roll your shoulders up towards your ears; keep them up and roll them back; keep them back and roll them down. That's the Roll and the Drop. You should feel the muscles under your armpits engage and your chest lift in front.
- To Lock, continue to press your shoulders down and scoop your elbows forward until they are in line with the seam on the side of your shirt along your rib cage. When you do the Lock phase, you will feel your abdominals engage to tilt your pelvis into a neutral position with your tailbone pointing downward.
- Once you've done the Roll-Drop-Lock, you can relax your arms but maintain the engagement of your upper back and abdominals. In this position, your neck and chest will be open and relaxed and your lower back and rear end will be relaxed. Practice until you can do the motion easily.

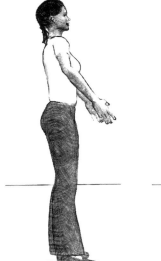 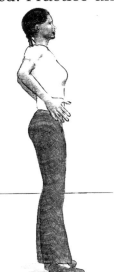 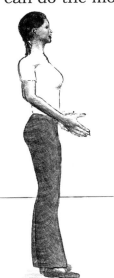 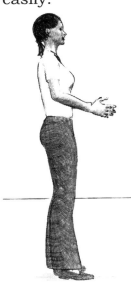

Roll shoulders up   *Roll shoulders back*   *Drop shoulders down*   *Lock torso into neutral*

Roll-Drop-Lock

DEEP BREATH

- Sit on a firm chair with your feet on the floor and your back against the chair back (place a book or block of wood under your feet if you can't touch the floor). Place one palm on your chest with your thumb resting between your collar bones and place the other palm over your belly button. As you breathe, the hand over your chest should not move. The hand over your belly button will move in with your exhale and out with your inhale.

- Roll-Drop-Lock and relax your neck and shoulders. Look straight ahead. Let your shoulder blades drop down towards your hips. It helps to imagine heavy velvet curtains hanging off of each shoulder blade.

- Your breathing cycle should begin with a stabilizing exhale during which you pull your belly button in towards your spine. You should feel the curve in your lower back straighten so your lower back presses against the chair back. Exhale for a count of 6 or 7, trying to open your throat into an O shape while slowly releasing the air past your chest and through your open mouth. Feel your abdomen flatten towards your spine and press the air up and out of your lungs.

- The inhale is a passive movement — a release of the abdominal and chest muscles. Relax and let the diaphragm muscle create a vacuum, pulling new air in through your nose and down to the base of your lungs. Inhale for a count of 3 or 4, allowing your diaphragm to press downward and outward to create space for your lungs to fill. Your tummy will expand outward as you do this.

- Practice this breathing pattern daily imagining your breath as a rolling wave.

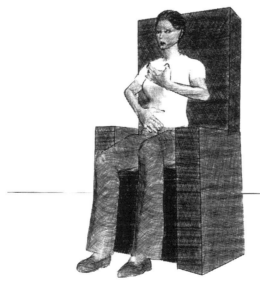

Deep Breath

SNOW ANGEL ARM RAISE WITH DEEP BREATH

- Stand with your back against a wall and equal weight over both feet. Roll-Drop-Lock. Relax your shoulders, and let your hands hang down by your sides with your palms facing forward and the backs of your arms and hands touching the wall. Your pinkies will be next to your hips.
- Visualize your arms as levers attached to pivot points at your shoulder blades. As with the deep breath exercise, you will begin your breathing cycle with an exhale, and because you are taking your hands overhead, the rules of engagement apply. Exhale, pull your belly button in, and drop your shoulder blades down while slowly raising your hands out to the sides and overhead in a smooth arc. Relax the tops of your shoulders and neck as you imagine that helium balloons attached to your thumbs are sliding them along the wall and lifting them up over your head. As your arms flow overhead, your shoulder blades should scoop out away from your spine.
- Your goal is to keep the backs of your arms and hands touching the wall so you can feel your shoulder blades' downward and outward scooping motion against the wall. But if your arms or the backs of your hands don't touch the wall, don't worry. Just press your back against the wall and let your arms flow in an arc. If you cannot get your hands all the way overhead, don't worry about that either. Take them as high as your weakest shoulder can go so you keep both sides of your body aligned. These things will improve as your range of motion improves.
- Inhale and let your tummy expand outward as you slowly lower your arms back down through the arc to your sides, scooping your shoulder blades back in toward your spine. Release any tension in the top of your shoulders and neck.
- Repeat 8-12 times.

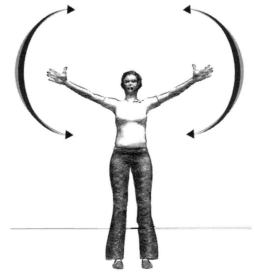

Snow Angel Arm Raise

Posture Walking

- Before you begin any strength-training workout, it is important to get your blood flowing. Walking is an excellent way to accomplish this.

- Roll-Drop-Lock, then start walking at a pace that allows you to carry on a conversation but not so slow that you could sing a song. As you walk, focus on correct posture — shoulders level over your hips, head balanced, front of your rib cage lifted, and pelvis in a neutral position. Your abdominals should be slightly contracted and your shoulder blades pulled downward.

- Look out about 10 feet in front of you and walk with confidence. To avoid throwing your body forward or using momentum to move, keep your body tall and think about bending and lifting one knee then extending that leg in front of you. With your back foot still on the floor, bend the back knee so you can touch the front heel down on the floor. Focus on stable placement of the heel.

- Make sure that leg is stable, then shift your center of gravity forward over the new foot to bring the toes down. Once you are stable over the new foot, roll through the balls of your toes on the back foot and push off, bringing it through to the front by bending and lifting the knee, extending your leg, and shifting onto that foot's heel.

- When you are striding fluidly, add Deep Breaths using the Snow Angel Arm Raise. Start with your hands down by your hips, palms facing forward, shoulders pressing down. Exhale and move your shoulder blades to sweep your hands in an arc, out to the sides and up overhead. Inhale as you lower your hands back to your sides following the same arc. Remember the Rules of Engagement! Pull that belly button in with your exhale as your hands go overhead.

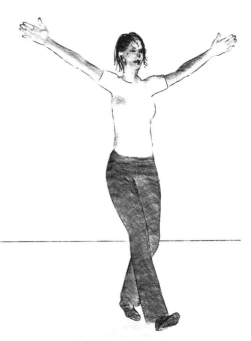

- After you've taken 10 to 20 deep breaths, you can add variety to your steps by walking on your toes, taking giant steps, or stepping diagonally. Let your arms flow with the legs for balance and be sure to maintain good posture with all strides.

- Your walking warm-up will last 5 to 10 minutes, at which time you should begin to break a sweat and breathe heavier.

Posture Walking

SPINE AND TORSO STRENGTH TRAINING

Exercises to strengthen the muscles surrounding the spine are essential for managing osteoporosis. As these muscles get stronger, your posture and movement will improve. Over time, your bones will strengthen.

In the **BONES** Lifestyle program, you do not have to get down on the floor to strengthen your muscles and bones or to improve your posture. The exercises in this book are safe and effective and these spine and torso exercises can be done while standing or sitting. If done consistently, they will build excellent posture, strength, and balance.

There are some floor exercises that ease the load on the muscles in your back, help develop better posture and strengthen your abdominal, hip, shoulder, arm, and thigh muscles. Pilates, yoga, and classic calisthenics all incorporate these exercises. But I have found that many of my clients have a difficult time sitting or lying on the floor, and even more have a hard time getting up off the floor. Furthermore, studies show that a significantly higher number of vertebral compression fractures occur in patients who performed flexion exercises (forward bending) compared to those who did extension exercises (straightening and lengthening the spine). Many of the common floor exercises in Pilates, yoga, and calisthenics involve trunk flexion. Trunk extension and upright exercises are much more appropriate for people with osteoporosis.

As you are doing the spine and torso exercises, keep in mind that it is the muscles that attach to the spine, rib cage, and pelvis that we are working on. You should feel those muscles engaging and your core abdominal muscles stabilizing, not your neck and the tops of your shoulders. The neck and shoulder muscles fall into the category that I call "bully muscles." They want to have all the fun and try to do the work the other muscles are supposed to do. When these bully muscles take over, the other muscles can't engage correctly. Focus on relaxing your neck and the tops of your shoulders as you engage the muscles around your rib cage, pelvis, and spine. To do this, breathe slow, deep breaths, and think about the muscles you should be engaging. Notice how they feel when engaged and then how they feel when released. Do not add resistance to your exercises until you can feel the correct muscles engaging and releasing on every repetition — otherwise the bullies will push their way into the game.

PELVIC TILT

- Stand with your feet hip-width apart, toes and knees facing forward. Roll-Drop-Lock. Relax your arms and rest your hands on the top crest of your pelvis. Your thumbs should be in back, along the top of the prominent pelvic bones and your pointer fingers should rest on the bones in the front.
- Bring your pelvis into a neutral position by tilting it forward or back until the thumbs and fingers are at the same height. Think of your pelvis being shaped like a bowl of pancake batter with your fingers on the bowl's rim. In a neutral position the bowl is sitting flat as if it were resting on the counter. Keep your shoulder blades pulled together and down, your chest lifted and open, and your spine tall throughout this exercise.
- Inhale and tilt your pelvis forward, lifting your tailbone as if you were pouring the pancake batter onto the griddle. In this position, your fingers in the front will be lower than your thumbs in the back. Exhale and scoop your tailbone under bringing the pelvis back to a neutral position as if placing your bowl on the counter. Repeat 8 to 12 times, inhaling as you pour the batter out, exhaling as you set the bowl on the counter.
- Next, with your hands still resting on the top crest of your pelvis, tip your pelvic bowl in a full circle as if you are trying to coat all the sides of your bowl with batter. Circle 8 to 12 times clockwise, then circle 8 to 12 times counterclockwise. As you circle your hips, focus on engaging your abdominal muscles and relaxing your rear end, shoulders, and neck. Keep your ribs and arms still.

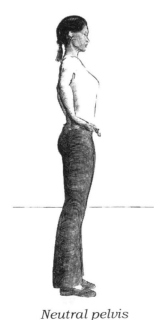

Neutral pelvis

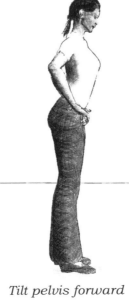

Tilt pelvis forward

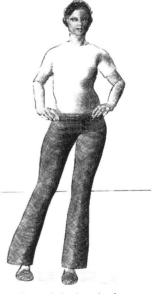

Tilt pelvis in circle

Pelvic Tilt

SHOULDER BLADE RETRACTION

- This movement originates in your upper back around your shoulder blades.
- Stand with your feet hip-width apart, toes and knees facing forward. Stabilize your spine with a Roll-Drop-Lock. Bend your elbows to bring your hands up in front of your chest and interlace your fingers. Rotate your palms so they face away from your body. Straighten your elbows and pull your shoulder blades down to drop your shoulders down away from your ears.
- If you feel any pain, modify the position by keeping your palms facing toward you, by bending your elbows, or by lowering your arms. Whichever position you use, be sure to keep your pelvis neutral.
- Relax your neck and the tops of your shoulders and imagine you have an orange between your shoulder blades.
- Exhale, pull your bellybutton in and squeeze your shoulder blades together — pulling them back and in toward your spine to press the orange juice out of the orange. Bend your elbows to bring your hands to your chest as you squeeze your shoulder blades together.
- Inhale and exhale again while you hold the contraction for 3 to 5 seconds to wring out all of the orange juice. As you do this, you will feel your chest muscles and the front of your shoulders stretch. Remember the First Rule of Engagement – pull your belly button in and be careful not to arch your lower back or throw your chest forward as you squeeze your upper back muscles.
- After 3 to 5 seconds, inhale and release the contraction, separating your shoulder blades by pushing your palms out in front of your body at shoulder height.
- Repeat this movement 8 to 12 times, holding each contraction for 3 to 5 seconds. You should feel your shoulder blades slide together when your hands come toward your body, then open out to the sides as your hands move away from your body.

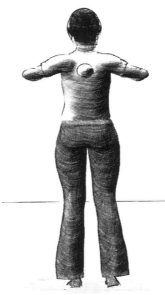

Position of imaginary orange

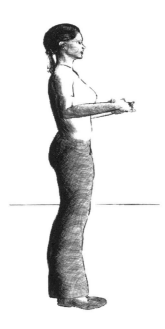

Interlace fingers

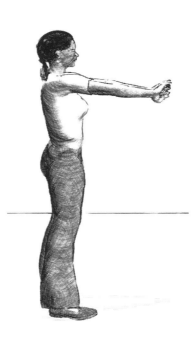

Separate shoulder blades

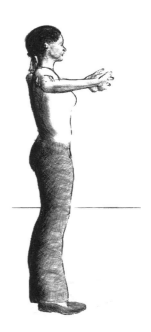

Squeeze shoulder blades together

Shoulder Blade Retraction

UPRIGHT ROW

- Stand with your weight evenly placed over both feet and Roll-Drop-Lock. Allow your arms to hang down by your sides, palms facing the sides of your thighs.
- Imagine hot air balloons are tied to each elbow and are lifting them out to the sides and up towards the sky. As your elbows lift, bend them, drop your shoulders, and slide your hands up your sides towards your armpits. Keep your neck and shoulders relaxed and exhale as you lift, then inhale as you slowly lower your hands back down to your sides. If you feel like a gorilla scratching his armpits, you are doing it correctly! Repeat this motion 8 to 12 times.
- Next, rotate your palms to face the fronts of your thighs, resting your hands against your thighs. Drop your shoulders. Lift and bend your elbows out to the sides and upwards again, this time sliding your hands up the front of your body towards your chest. When your elbows are even with your shoulders, make sure your shoulders and neck are relaxed then squeeze your shoulder blades together as you did in the Shoulder Blade Retraction exercise. Remember the Rules of Engagement — exhale and pull your belly button in as you engage your upper back muscles. Then inhale and slide your hands back down to the start position. Repeat 8 to 12 times.
- As you get stronger and can do this exercise without hunching your shoulders or tightening your neck, add 1 to 8 pound hand weights to this movement. Hold onto the weights gently then slide your hands up your body.

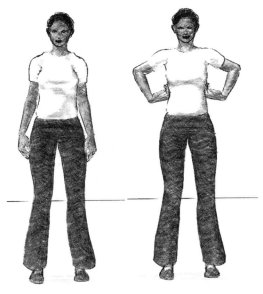

Palms face side
of thighs   Palms to armpits

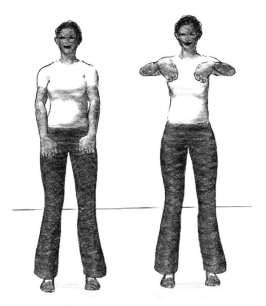

Palms face front   Palms to chest
of thighs

Upright Row

Pulling The Horse's Reigns

- Sit toward the front of a hard seat with your back tall and chin lifted. Keep one knee bent with the foot flat on the floor. Extend the other knee so your heel rests on the floor out in front of you. Roll-Drop-Lock.
- With your palms facing each other, reach your arms out over the extended leg, tilting your pelvic bowl forward to bring your chest over your thighs. You are not trying to touch your toes. Just tilt your pelvis and torso forward on a diagonal a few inches, keeping your back flat and your chest open and lifted.
- Then tip your pelvic bowl back to neutral to bring your torso upright. As you tilt upright, pull your belly button in and squeeze your shoulder blades together while sliding your elbows behind your torso as if you are pulling a horse's reigns to stop him. Inhale as you tilt forward and exhale as you sit upright. Keep your torso stable and your shoulders and neck relaxed throughout the movement. Be careful not to arch your lower back.
- Once you can do this movement with a flat back and relaxed shoulders and neck, add a resistance exercise band (the band can be flat or round). Place the band under the arch of your extended leg's foot and gently hold onto both ends of the band, one end in each hand. If it's more comfortable, you can wrap the band ends around your wrists.
- Repeat the exercise 8 to 12 times on each leg.

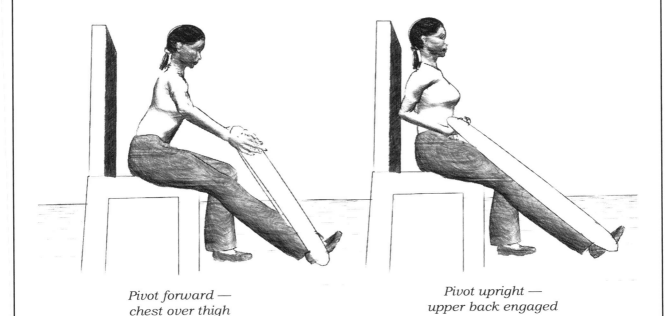

Pivot forward —
chest over thigh

Pivot upright —
upper back engaged

Pulling The Horse's Reigns

HIP AND LEG STRENGTH TRAINING

As the exercises get more complex, the Rules of Engagement become even more important. Even though you are focusing on your lower body in these exercises, the Rules of Engagement still apply — Roll–Drop–Lock before each exercise to bring your shoulder girdle and pelvic girdle into a neutral position so your spine is stable. Until this stabilization becomes a habit, you may need to Roll–Drop–Lock every few repetitions.

Your knees should not hurt when you do these exercises. To protect your knees, always keep your knees in line over your heels. On lunges and steps, the knee of the front stepping leg should not extend forward over your toes as this puts a tremendous load on your knee joint. On the Squat, Reverse Squat, Toe Raises and Jumps, neither knee should extend forward. When you are doing the leg exercises, pause periodically to look down at your feet. If you can see your entire foot then your knee(s) are correctly aligned. If not, push your hips backward and bend your knees until your legs are in correct alignment.

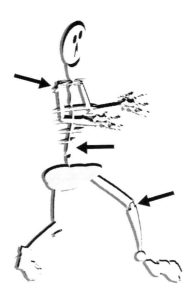

When you are doing the hip and leg exercises, focus on engaging your upper back and core muscles and keep your knee(s) aligned over your heel(s).

BACK LUNGE

- This is the easiest lunge to do. It's basically a giant step backwards, but don't try to rush through it using momentum. Use your muscles and feel your body move slowly and fluidly.
- Start with your feet side by side, weight equally placed over both feet. Roll-Drop-Lock to stabilize your spine. Shift your center of gravity over one foot and let your arms float up in front of your chest for balance. Keep your chin lifted and your torso straight as you lift the other knee to bring your foot off the floor. Then reach the lifted foot as far behind you as you can while allowing your torso to tilt forward and your arms to straighten slightly for counterbalance.
- Feel the floor under your toes to be sure you have a stable base. As your back foot touches the floor, allow the back knee to bend but keep the back heel lifted. Pull your belly button in to tilt your pelvis into a neutral position and slowly shift your center of gravity back over the balls of the toes on the back foot. Remember, your front knee should be lined up over the heel, not pushed forward over the toes. If you look down and can see your whole front foot, you are doing it correctly.
- To return to start position, Roll-Drop-Lock, engaging your core abdominals and upper back muscles, and imagine that your leg muscles are springs. Bend both knees, lower your hips toward the floor a little and push off the balls of your toes on the back foot, bringing the knee up and forward. Set your foot down in the start position.
- Repeat 8 to 12 times on each foot. You can alternate feet or repeat a full set on one foot, followed by a full set on the other foot.

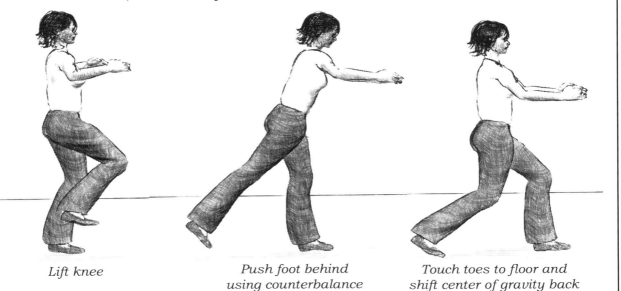

Lift knee   *Push foot behind using counterbalance*   *Touch toes to floor and shift center of gravity back*

Back Lunge

FORWARD LUNGE

- This is basically a giant step forward. As with the Back Lunge, it is important to use your muscles to create the movement, not momentum, so move slowly and deliberately, bending and straightening your joints.
- Start with your feet side by side. Roll-Drop-Lock. Rest your hands on the top crest of your hips or let them hang by your sides. If you prefer to hold your arms out to the sides for balance, that is fine.
- Shift your center of gravity over one foot, and bring the other knee up in front of your body to lift that foot off the floor. Then extend your lifted knee and reach your lifted heel as far in front of you as you can.
- Bend the back knee and shift your center of gravity forward to bring the front heel to the floor in a giant step. As you do this, your back heel will roll up off the floor.
- With both knees bent, lower your front toes down onto the floor and shift your center of gravity forward a bit more until it is centered between your feet. You should feel stable in this position with your front toes and heel securely on the floor, your back knee bent, and your back toes pushing down into the floor. Check to make sure your front knee is aligned over your heel — can you see your entire front foot? If not, shift your hips backwards until you can.
- To return to the starting position, Roll-Drop-Lock and scoop your pelvis under to engage your core muscles. Press your back toes downward, and bring your back knee forward slightly to engage your thigh muscles. Then simply move your center of gravity backwards and roll the back heel down. Lift your front knee to bring the front foot off the floor as your center of gravity shifts backward. Lower the front foot down to the floor next to the other one.
- An alternative option is to continue moving forward. To get out of the lunge this way, start as you did before and step into a forward lunge but instead of lifting the front foot and bringing it back next to the back foot, spring off the back foot and bring it forward next to the front foot the same way you did to get out of the back lunge. You will end the lunge a giant step forward.
- If you have the space, you may choose to continue moving forward by bringing the back leg through and stepping into a new lunge rather than stopping with your feet side by side. Many people find this continuous movement easier. Just remember to use your muscles. Don't let momentum carry you through with poor form.
- Lunge forward 8 to 12 times on each leg.

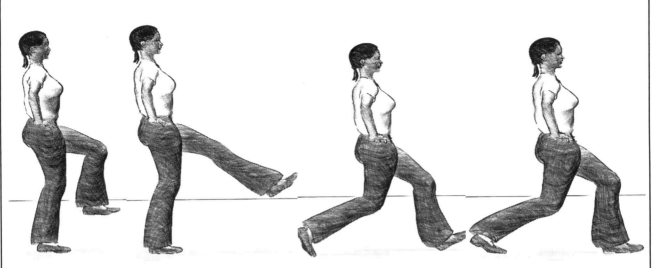

| Lift knee | Reach heel out in front | Shift center of gravity forward | Bring front toes down to floor |

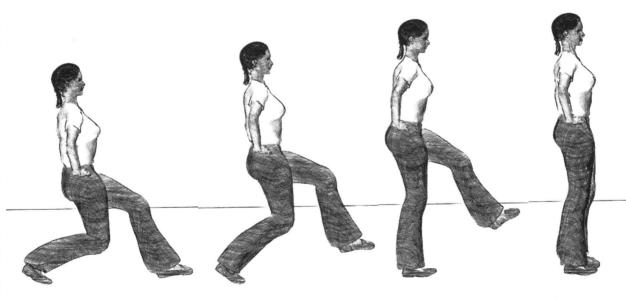

| Scoop pelvis | Shift center of gravity backwards to lift front foot | Roll back heel down | Bring front foot back and step down |

Forward Lunge

SIDE LUNGE

- Like the other lunges, this lunge is a giant step. But this time you are step-ping to the side. It's amazing how many people feel uncomfortable stepping to the side, so to avoid doing it, they turn their pelvis, twist their spine, and step forward. The problem is, there are times when you must step out to the side and if you've never practiced it correctly, your muscles won't know what to do and you may injure your hip, knee, ankle, and/or back. As with the other exercises, practice using your muscles to control the movement.

- Start with your feet side by side. Roll-Drop-Lock to stabilize your spine. Look at a point on the wall out in front of you. You will keep your head, pelvis, and rib cage facing that point throughout the exercise. The key to a good side lunge is to focus your mind on your center of gravity.

- With your knees softly bent, shift your center of gravity over one foot. Lift the other foot off the floor, bringing that knee up in front of your body. Keep your center of gravity stable over the standing foot. Think about the outside of the ankle on your lifted foot, and slowly move it out to the side. Only move it as far to the side as you comfortably can. If you are uncom-fortable doing this, hold onto something and practice this motion a few times before moving on.

- When the lifted foot is out to the side, touch the big toe to the floor. Then, with both knees bent, push your hips back and shift your center of gravity sideways, over the stepping foot, bringing the rest of the toes and heel onto the floor. Keep your toes and knees facing forward and your hips back to keep the stepping knee aligned over the heel.

- To get out of the side lunge, Roll-Drop-Lock and shift your hips back to the center so your weight is evenly distributed over both feet. Continue shifting your center of gravity until it is back in line over the initial stand-ing leg, then lift the stepping foot up off the floor. Straighten your body to an upright position and bring your lifted foot down to the floor beside the other foot.

- Repeat 8 to 12 times on each leg.

- As your strength and balance develop, start taking larger steps to the side. Then, with both knees bent, spring off the stepping leg as you shift your center of gravity through the center and come up to balance over the standing leg.

> **Safety Note:** *It is important to move with your joints on this exercise. Don't lift your leg so high to the side that you have to tip your body to accommodate it. Lift the knee in front of you, then slide the foot to the side before you shift your weight. If you're at risk for osteoporosis in your hips, this will protect a fragile femoral neck (the section of the thigh bone that attaches to the pelvis).*

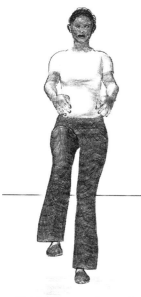

*Shift center of gravity
and lift leg*

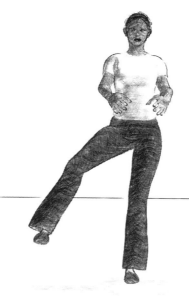

Move leg to side

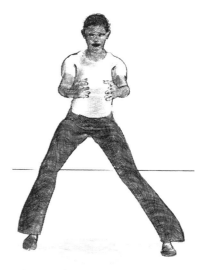

*Step down and shift
center of gravity*

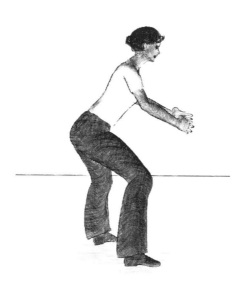

Side View

Side Lunge

STEP

- The purpose of this step exercise is not aerobic training but strength training. Good form is important, and the more controlled you do it, the better. Try to step quietly, so your feet don't make any sound as you make contact with the step or floor.
- Stand on the floor in front of a step with both feet flat on the floor and your hand on a hand rail or wall if you'd like. Roll-Drop-Lock.
- Shift your center of gravity over one foot then bend the other knee and lift it up in front of you. Extend the lifted leg slightly at the knee so your foot is lined up over the step.
- While standing upright, place your heel down onto the step first, then roll your toes down so the entire foot is on the step. Your lifted knee should be aligned over the front heel when your foot is on the step. Keep your weight over the back (lower) leg.
- Roll onto the toes of your back foot to lift that heel off the floor, and bring the knee of that leg forward into a small bend so your leg has a springiness to it. You should feel your toes pushing down into the floor. This leg will be the spring that pushes you up onto the step. Bend the back knee a little farther, push your hips back, and bring your chest forward slightly in counterbalance.
- Spring off the lower leg, pushing off the floor to bring that foot up while at the same time bending that knee and hip to bring the foot forward. As you bring the lower knee up, straighten your torso, lining up your pelvis under your shoulders. Place the springing foot on the step next to the other foot.
- To step back down to the floor, shift your center of gravity over one leg and lift the other knee to bring its foot up off the step.
- Move the lifted foot behind you, and lower your toes slowly to the floor. As you reach for the floor behind you, bring your chest slightly forward in counterbalance. Once you can feel the floor under your toes, begin to shift your center of gravity back over that foot. Gently lower your weight and put your heel down. Tilt your torso upright and bring the other foot down to the floor.
- When you step up, place your heel on the step first. When you step down, touch your toes to the floor first. Step up and down 8 to 12 times with the right foot and 8 to 12 times with the left foot.
- If necessary, look down at the step during the first few repetitions to check for correct foot placement on the center of the step, then look up and trust your muscles to remember your foot placement. Never put your full weight onto the step or floor until you feel support under your foot. Be careful to keep your front knee lined up over your heel. Focus on the muscles in the calves, thighs, and rear end that are lifting and lowering your body.

Step Up Heel First

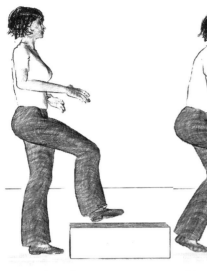
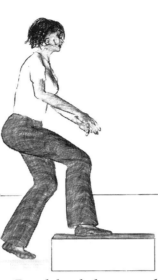
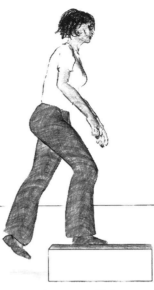
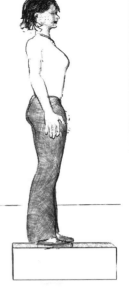

Bring foot over step   *Bend back knee and lift back heel*   *Spring up off floor*   *Bring foot onto step*

Step Down Toe First

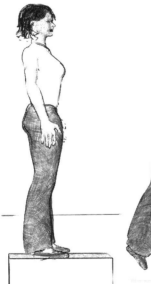
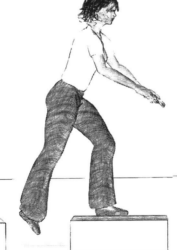
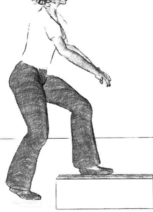
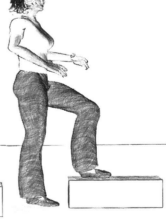

Shift center of gravity   *Reach toes to floor*   *Shift weight back and down*   *Straighten torso*

Step

SQUAT

- The most important part of the squat is to push your hips back and keep your knees aligned over your heels. You will use counterbalance to achieve this.
- Stand with the backs of your calves or knees touching the seat of a chair. Your feet should be parallel, about hip-width apart. Roll-Drop-Lock to stabilize your spine.
- Push your hips back and bend your knees as if you are going to sit down. The backs of your legs should remain in contact with the chair throughout the entire exercise. Don't try to sit all the way down. Start by pushing your hips back about an inch.
- Keep your upper back and abdominal muscles engaged and bring your chest and arms forward in counterbalance, tilting your torso into a diagonal position as you push your hips back into the squat. By bringing your arms up in front of you, they will help you balance.
- Glance down at your feet — you should be able to see your entire foot. If you can't, or you don't feel the chair behind your legs, it means your knees have shifted forward, and you are placing too much strain on your knee joints. In the correct position, you will be using your thigh muscles and counterbalance to relieve the strain from your knees and back.
- Once you feel the coordination of the hips and knees, you can push your hips farther back. Remember, your chest is your counterbalance so if you push your hips back farther, you must also bring your chest farther forward.
- When you are comfortable with the hips back/chest forward position, you can start lowering your bottom towards the floor after you've pushed your hips back. Keep your calves touching the chair behind you so you will know if you move your knees forward. Push your hips back, then lower your bottom an inch or two towards the chair seat but don't sit all the way down.
- To return to standing, pull your belly button in and up, and slide your hips forward as you straighten your knees.
- When you are confident that your form is correct, you can move away from the chair to do your squats. When you are down in the squat, you should be looking at the floor about five feet in front of you so your neck stays in line with the rest of your spine.
- If your back hurts when you perform a squat, check to make sure you are bending your knees, and make sure you have engaged your core correctly by redoing the Roll-Drop-Lock. Do not lower your hips below the level of your knees.
- Repeat 8 to 12 times.

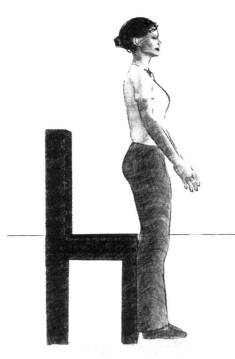

Calves touch chair

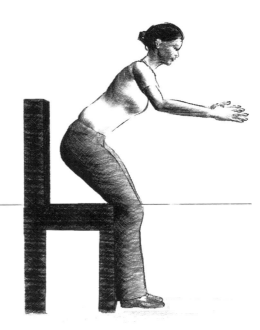

Press hips back and bend knees

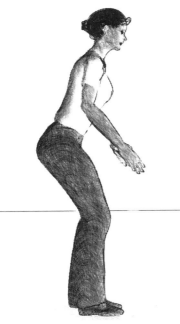

Knees align over heels

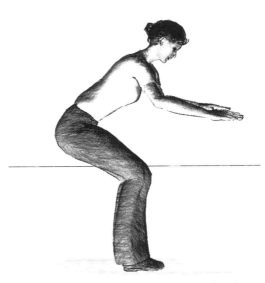

Continue to press hips back and lower bottom

Squat

REVERSE SQUAT/CHAIR RAISE

- A major goal of this exercise is to feel how physics makes movement easier. When you use the principle of counterbalance, standing up from a chair is simple.
- Start in a seated position on a bench, chair, or exercise ball. Place your feet flat on the floor with the tops of your thighs facing up towards the ceiling and your knees hip-width apart so your toes and knees face forward. Roll-Drop-Lock to stabilize your spine, then reach your arms out in front of your body for counterbalance.
- Keeping your belly button in and your back flat, bring your chest forward over your knees (think "nose over toes") until your bottom lifts up off the chair. At this point, push your heels into the floor, exhale and think about lifting your belly button up. Pull your arms down to your sides as you slide your hips forward, straightening your body to a standing position. Your pelvis will slide forward under your chest as you move upright. As with a squat, keep your knees relaxed and aligned over your heels. Don't lock your knees by overextending them.
- Return to the seat in the same manner that you did in the squat — touch the backs of your calves against the chair, push your hips back, bring your chest forward, and bend your knees around the chair seat. Slowly lower your bottom all the way down to the chair, then tilt your torso to an upright position over your pelvis. Control your body as you lower; do not just plop back down onto the chair.
- The goal is to complete this movement without pushing up off the chair with your hands, but if you need assistance, you can place your hands on the seat for support.
- Repeat 8 to 12 times.

> ## Bench, Chair, or Ball?
> *The technique to stand up is the same if you use a chair, bench, or exercise ball. A firmer surface is easier but as you advance, you can use an exercise ball or soft sofa.*
>
> *Do NOT use an exercise ball without a spotter if you haven't done it before as they can be very unstable. Place the ball on a carpeted surface and near a wall for support if needed. To sit down on the ball, have your spotter hold it still or stabilize it with one hand and lower down carefully so the ball doesn't roll out from under you.*

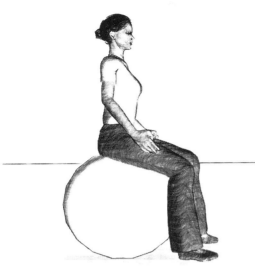

*Sit upright over the center
of a ball or chair*

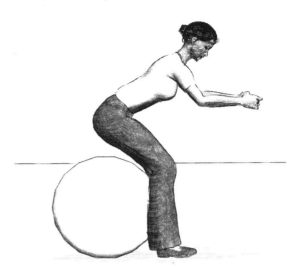

*Nose Over Toes
Bring chest and arms forward*

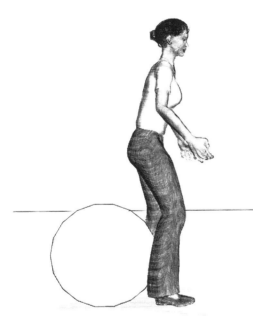

Slide hips forward and stand upright

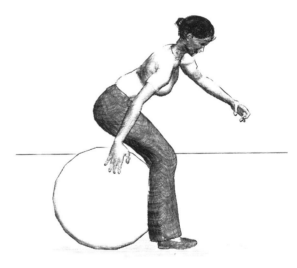

*To sit down, stabilize ball if using
one, push hips back and bring chest
forward*

Reverse Squat

TOE RAISES AND JUMPING

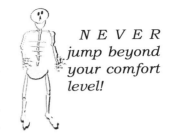

N E V E R jump beyond your comfort level!

- Roll-Drop-Lock. Shift your hips back, bring your chest forward, and bend your knees into a mini-squat (make sure you can see your entire foot). It helps to use your arms for counterbalance as you learn this movement, so bring your hands out in front of your body. If you feel like you are downhill skiing then you are in a good position.

- Before jumping, you will want to practice toe raises (also called faux jumps). Engage your abdominals, pull your hands down by your sides, and slide your hips forward, stacking your shoulders over your pelvis. Continue moving your pelvis forward another inch to lift your heels off the floor and roll up onto the balls of your toes. At this point your shoulders will be in line over your pelvis, knees, and toes. Balance for a few seconds with your heels lifted, then drop your heels to the floor, 'plopping' them down to the ground as you lower back into a mini-squat.

- One cycle includes 5 to 10 toe raises, with a pause in between each one. If you haven't jumped before or are just getting started with the exercises, do toe raises until you feel balanced and in complete control. If you have any discomfort, pain, active fractures, or other limitations just stick with toe raises. You will still obtain benefits.

- When you are ready to progress to the jump, stand with your feet parallel about shoulder-width apart. Roll-Drop-Lock and lower into a deeper squat allowing your arms to extend out in front of your body. To jump, push your hips forward as you press your hands down by your sides. Push up and off the ground, straightening your legs and rolling through your feet. You don't need to jump high to get adequate impact on the landing.

- When landing, cushion your body by landing on your toes then rolling your heels down while pushing your hips back into a squat. Because you will be bending at the ankle, knee and hip, you will reduce the chance of injury while gaining the benefits of the jump. Think of yourself as a spring coiling in the squat, uncoiling as you jump, then recoiling into another squat.

- Repeat a cycle of 5 to 10 jumps, pausing between each jump. Do a total of 1 to 10 cycles depending on your fitness and comfort level.

> *The key to successful impact for bone building is to pause between the toe raises or jumps and keep your body aligned and stable.*

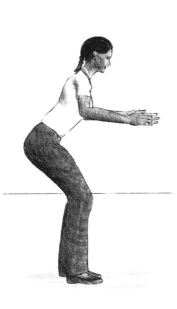
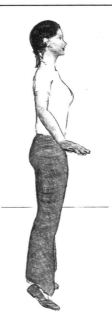
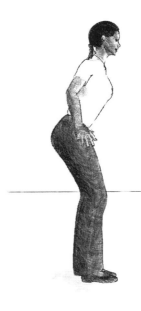

Shift hips back into a mini-squat

Press hands down and pull hips forward raising onto toes

Plop heels down and push hips back

Toe Raises

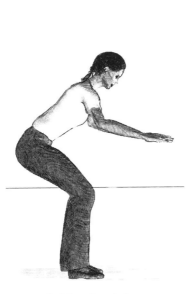
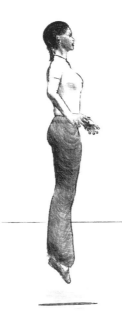
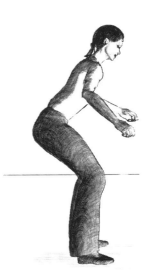

Push hips back into a squat

Push hands down, pull hips forward, and spring off the ground

Bend ankles, knees, and hips on landing

Jumps

WRIST EXERCISES

The third part of the body where we need bone–building exercise is in the wrists. As mentioned earlier, the bones with the greatest percentage of trabecular tissue tend to be the first ones affected by osteoporosis. The vertebra, femoral neck, and wrist are all high in trabecular bone and are the most common sites of osteoporotic fracture. When you are ready to add resistance to your exercise routine, adding hand weights or exercise bands to your other exercises will add resistance for your wrists as well. But remember to keep your wrists stable when you are holding something so you don't strain them. The exercises in this section will cause the muscles to tug the bones in your wrists in all directions.

Wrist Circles
- This exercise can be done while seated in a chair, while standing up, or while doing balance exercises.
- Roll-Drop-Lock to stabilize your spine. Relax your neck. Grip a pencil in your fingers as if you were going to write. Imagine you are in front of a big, blank wall.
- Holding the pencil out in front of your chest, draw a circle on that imaginary wall by moving your wrist in a circle. Your forearm will rotate with your wrist but be careful, your shoulder and elbow will try to do the motion for your wrist. Stabilize them by bringing your elbow in to the side of your rib cage so it can't move. Watch the shape your hand draws and strive for a precise, smooth, round circle.
- Draw 10 circles in each direction then repeat with the other hand. As you get good at drawing circles, add figure 8's and alphabet letters.

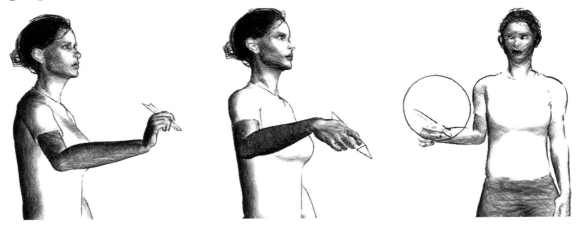

Wrist Circles

PLAY THE PIANO

- Sit or stand with your feet parallel and a little wider than hip-width apart. Roll-Drop-Lock and let your arms hang in front of your body, palms facing your thighs. Bend your elbows so your hands are in front of you, palms down as if your hands are resting on piano keys. This is a neutral wrist position.
- Keep your torso upright and neck and shoulders relaxed. If this position causes discomfort in your neck, shoulders, or hands, you can rest your hands on a tabletop or on your thighs.
- With your palms facing down, turn both wrists out to the sides, moving your thumbs outward, away from the center.
- Then turn both wrists inward, bringing your thumbs toward your belly button. Keep your palms facing down throughout the movement.
- To keep this movement in your wrists, not your elbows and shoulders, imagine you are holding a water bottle under each armpit. When you move your wrists outward, your goal is to bring the pinkies closer to the outside of your forearm. When you bring your wrists inward, bring the thumbs closer to the inside of your forearms.
- Repeat in both directions 8 to 12 times.

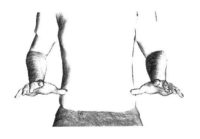
Wrists neutral

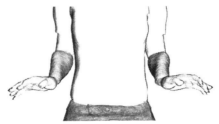
Wrists turn out

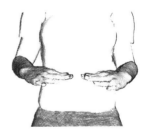
Wrists turn in

Play The Piano

WRIST HYPEREXTENSION

- Sit or stand with your feet parallel and a little wider than hip-width apart. Roll-Drop-Lock and let your arms hang down in front of your body, palms facing your thighs.
- **Press Forward:** Bend your elbows to bring your hands up to chest height, palms facing the floor. When your hands reach chest height, turn your fingertips up toward the ceiling.
  - With your palms facing away from your body, press the base of your palms straight out in front of your chest, straightening your elbows. When fully extended, your arms will be at shoulder height with your wrists bent back and your fingertips pointed up as if you were pushing against a wall in front of you. Focus on pressing the base of your palms away from your body to get full hyperextension of the wrists.
  - Then relax your wrists allowing your palms to face the floor. Without tightening your neck or the tops of your shoulders, slide your elbows back along your sides to bring your hands back towards your chest.
- **Press To The Sides:** Next, from the position in front of your chest, pull your fingertips up again and rotate your shoulders outward so your palms face to the side.
  - Imagine you are in a narrow hallway and push your palms outward as if you are pushing the base of your palms against the walls beside you.
  - Relax your wrists and bring your elbows back in beside your rib cage.
- **Press Down:** Relax your arms and let them hang down beside your thighs with your palms rotated to face behind you.
  - Lift your elbows up behind you so your hands rest next to your waist. Your palms will still be facing behind you.
  - Pull your fingertips back, so your wrist is in hyperextension and your palms face the floor. Press the base of your palms down toward the floor as if you were pressing on a table, straightening your elbows.
  - Relax your wrists and let your arms hang by your sides.
  - Repeat the three motions (pressing to the front, to the sides, and down) 8 to 12 times.
  - To help keep your neck and the tops of your shoulders relaxed, imagine that your hands are the wings of a butterfly, gently fluttering with the movement of your arms. Because this motion requires you to engage your upper back muscles, you must follow the rules of engagement.

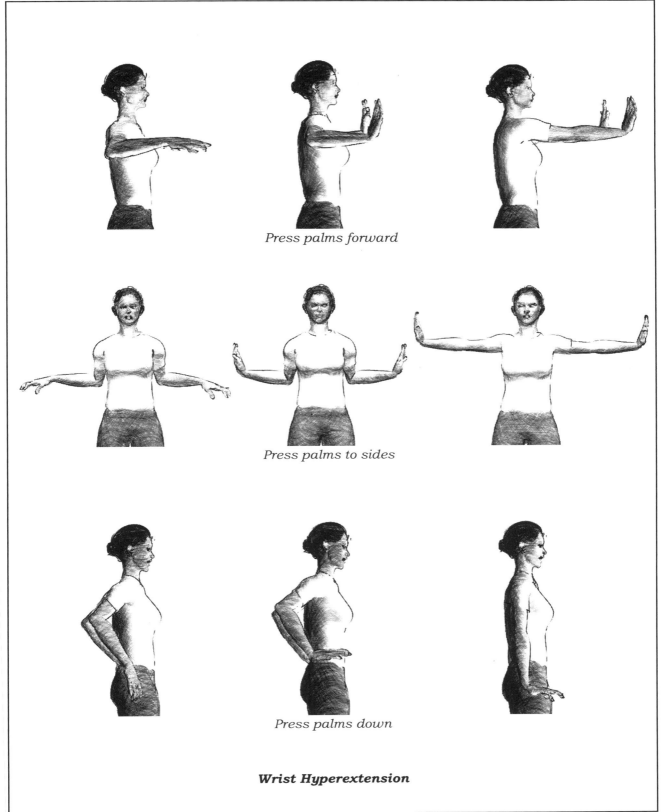

Press palms forward

Press palms to sides

Press palms down

Wrist Hyperextension

HOW TO

MODIFIED BONES LIFESTYLE
EXERCISE PROGRAM
FOR SEVERE OSTEOPOROSIS©

If you have been diagnosed with severe (also called advanced) osteoporosis, or have experienced a fragility fracture then follow these modifications for the **BONES** Lifestyle Workout. Read through each exercise carefully, then apply the modifications. Use a wall, counter or sturdy table, and a stable chair with armrests for the exercises. If you are new to exercise, experience any pain with the regular **BONES** Lifestyle Exercises, or if you are concerned about fracturing a bone, this is a good place to start.

If you do have severe osteoporosis, do these exercises with someone who can assist you and help you maintain good form, especially if you feel unsteady or are rehabilitating after a fracture. Don't be embarrassed or shy to ask for help from a physical therapist or a personal trainer. Take this book with you and show them the recommended exercises. They will evaluate your form and suggest safe alternatives if you have any pain or limitations.

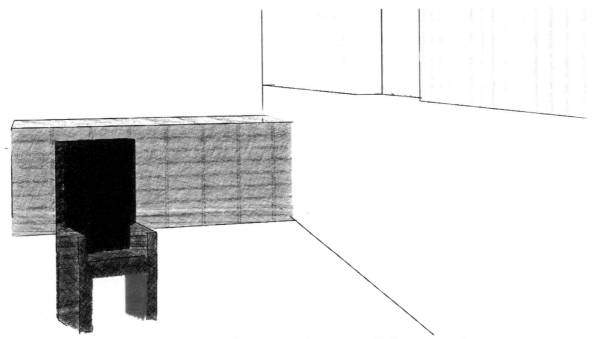

Use a sturdy chair, counter, or wall for support

MODIFIED WARM-UP FOR
SEVERE OSTEOPOROSIS

MODIFIED DEEP BREATH

- Sit on a firm chair with your feet on the floor and your back against the chair back (place a book or block of wood under your feet if you can't touch the floor). Place one palm on your chest with your thumb resting between your collar bones and place the other palm over your belly button. As you breathe, the hand over your chest should not move. The hand over your belly button will move in with your exhale and out with your inhale.
- Relax your neck and shoulders. Look straight ahead. Let your shoulder blades drop down towards your hips. It helps to imagine heavy velvet curtains hanging off of each shoulder blade.
- Your breathing cycle should begin with a stabilizing exhale during which you pull your belly button in towards your spine. You should feel the curve in your lower back straighten so your lower back presses against the chair back. Exhale for a count of 6 or 7, trying to open your throat into an O shape while slowly releasing the air past your chest and through your open mouth. Feel your abdomen flatten towards your spine and press the air up and out of your lungs.
- The inhale is a passive movement — a release of the abdominal and chest muscles. Relax and let the diaphragm muscle create a vacuum, pulling new air in through your nose and down to the base of your lungs. Inhale for a count of 3 or 4, allowing your diaphragm to press downward and outward to create space for your lungs to fill. Your tummy will expand outward as you do this.
- Practice this breathing pattern daily imagining your breath as a rolling wave.

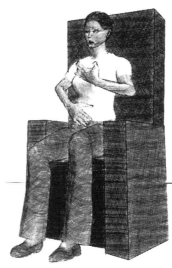

Modified Deep Breath

MODIFIED SNOW ANGEL ARM RAISE

- Stand with your back against a wall with equal weight over both feet or sit on a sturdy chair with both feet on the floor or a block. Relax your shoulders, and let your hands hang down by your sides with your palms facing forward and the backs of your arms and hands touching the wall. Your pinkies will be next to your hips.
- Visualize your arms as levers attached to pivot points at your shoulder blades. As with the Deep Breath exercise, you will begin your breathing cycle with an exhale, and because you are taking your hands overhead, the Rules of Engagement apply. Exhale, pull your belly button in, and drop your shoulder blades down while slowly raising your hands out to the sides and overhead in a smooth arc. Relax the tops of your shoulders and neck as you imagine that helium balloons attached to your thumbs are sliding them along the wall and lifting them up over your head. As your arms flow overhead, your shoulder blades should scoop out away from your spine.
- Your goal is to keep your back and the backs of your arms and hands touching the wall or chair back so you can feel your shoulder blades' downward and outward scooping motion. But if your arms or the backs of your hands don't touch the wall, don't worry. Just press your back against the wall or chair and let your arms flow in an arc. If you cannot get your hands all the way overhead, don't worry about that either. Take them as high as your weakest shoulder can go so you keep both sides of your body aligned. These things will improve as your range of motion improves.
- Inhale and let your tummy expand outward as you slowly lower your arms back down through the arc to your sides. Release any tension in the top of your shoulders and neck.
- Repeat 5 to 10 times.

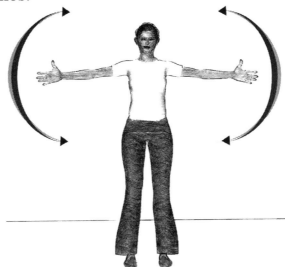

Modified Snow Angel

MODIFIED POSTURE WALKING

- Before you begin a strength-training workout, it is important to get your blood flowing. Walking is an excellent way to accomplish this.
- If you need assistance, use a walker or cane adjusted to your height so you remain upright. You can also walk on a treadmill set at a slow speed, or walk next to a wall or around a table resting one hand on it for support.
- Stand with your feet hip-width apart, toes and knees facing forward. Feel your balance evenly centered over both feet and keep your knees softly bent.
- To avoid leaning forward or using momentum to move, keep your body tall and think about bending and lifting one knee then extending that leg in front of you. Focus on placing your forward foot on the floor. With your back foot still on the floor, bend the back knee so you can touch the front heel down on the floor. Make sure that leg is stable, then shift your center of gravity forward over the new foot to bring the toes down. Once you are stable over the new foot, roll through the balls of your toes on the back foot and push off, bringing it through to the front by bending and lifting the knee, extending your leg, and shifting onto that foot's heel.
- Do not shuffle. Practice a full stride in which you pick your back foot up off the floor and move it forward instead of shuffling it along.
- As you walk, maintain correct posture — shoulders over your hips, chin level, front of your rib cage lifted and pelvis in a neutral position with your abdominal muscles engaged. Look out about 10 feet in front of you, and walk with confidence.
- Walk at a comfortable pace for 3 to 5 minutes.

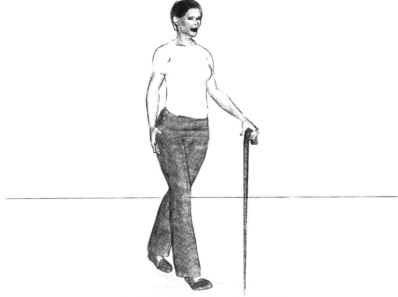

Modified Posture Walking

MODIFIED SPINE AND TORSO STRENGTH TRAINING FOR SEVERE OSTEOPOROSIS

Exercises to strengthen the muscles surrounding the spine are essential for managing osteoporosis. As these muscles get stronger, your posture and movement will improve, and over time, your bones will strengthen.

MODIFIED ROLL-DROP-LOCK

- Remember that your pelvis is shaped like a bowl. When your spine is in a neutral position, the bowl is sitting flat as if it were resting on the counter and your rib cage will sit flat over the top of the pelvic bowl like a cheese grater. This exercise will train your muscles to bring your spine into a neutral position so the rib cage and pelvis are both neutral and your spine is stable. You will notice that every exercise following this one reminds you to Roll-Drop-Lock because the movement sets up necessary support for your spine.
- Stand with your back against a wall or sit on a hard seat.
- Hunch your shoulders up to your ears then roll them back and down towards the floor (this is the "Roll" and the "Drop"). In this position, your shoulder blades will be pushing against the wall and your lower back will not be touching the wall.
- With your shoulders still pulled down, slide your elbows forward until they are even with the seam on the side of your shirt and at the same time pull your belly button in toward your spine, pressing your lower back toward the wall (this is the "Lock"). When you do this, your shoulder blades will flatten out. It's okay if your entire lower back doesn't contact the wall but you should feel your weight shift back slightly over your heels.
- Relax your arms so your hands hang down by the seam of your pants but maintain your pelvic–shoulder alignment. This is a neutral spine position.
- Repeat 5 to 10 times.
- Breathing helps with this movement — exhale as you drop your shoulders down and scoop your shoulders and pelvis forward. Inhale as your roll your shoulders up and back.
- The Roll-Drop-Lock is not a big movement — keep it controlled and precise and remember that the effort is in the shoulder girdle and abdominal muscles, not through the buttocks. As you get stronger and more comfortable with this movement, practice doing it away from a wall (holding onto a counter or table for support if needed).

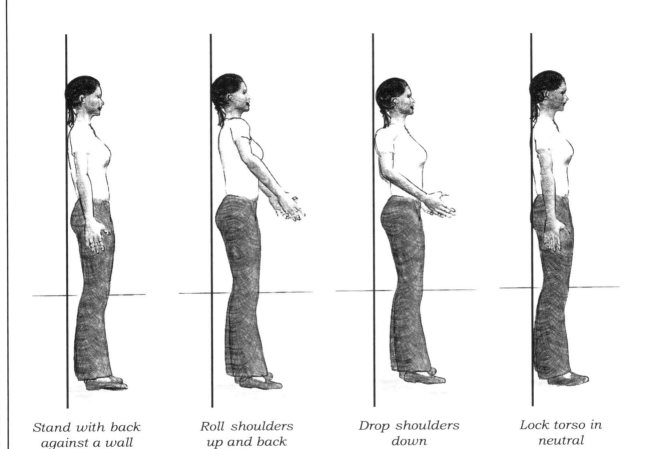

<table>
<tr>
<td>Stand with back
against a wall</td>
<td>Roll shoulders
up and back</td>
<td>Drop shoulders
down</td>
<td>Lock torso in
neutral</td>
</tr>
</table>

Modified Roll-Drop-Lock

Modified Chin Slide

- Lie on your bed with a pillow under your head or sit in a chair with a high back. Place a pillow behind your head so it rests between your head and the chair. Rest your hands beside you, on your thighs, or on the chair arms.
- Roll-Drop-Lock to stabilize your spine and relax your neck and shoulders. Gently press the back of your head straight back against the pillow, contracting the muscles in your neck and back.
- Notice that as you engage your neck and upper back muscles in this manner, your lower back comes slightly forward away from the chair or lifts slightly off the bed.
- Your head should move less than an inch. If it moves more, add another pillow.
- Release the contraction and recheck your postural alignment. Repeat 5 to 10 times, being careful to press the back of your head into the pillow. Don't tip your head back or forward.
- Keep the contraction very gentle and small.
- Never overstrain your neck.

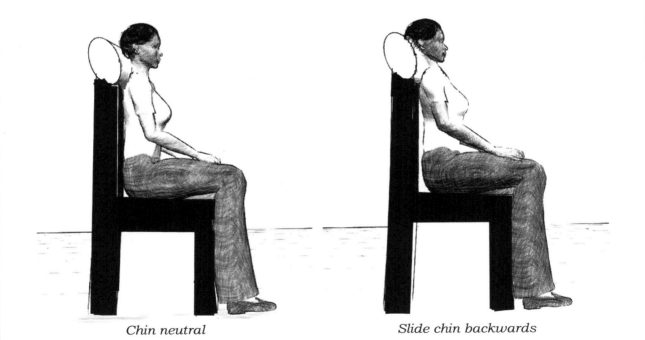

Chin neutral   *Slide chin backwards*

Modified Chin Slide

MODIFIED SHOULDER BLADE RETRACTION

- This movement originates in your upper back and shoulder blades. Stand with your back against a wall or sit in a chair with a hard back and seat. Let your arms hang by your sides.
- Roll-Drop-Lock to stabilize your spine. Relax your neck and the tops of your shoulders.
- Exhale and squeeze your shoulder blades together, pressing them back against the wall or chair and pulling them in together toward your spine. Your chest will lift as you do this movement.
- This is a focused movement of your upper back around the shoulder blades. Keep the movement small and remember the rules of engagement by pulling your belly button in as you squeeze your shoulder blades together. Don't arch your back or throw your chest forward.
- Hold the contraction for 3 to 5 seconds then release to separate your shoulder blades.
- Repeat 5 to 10 times.

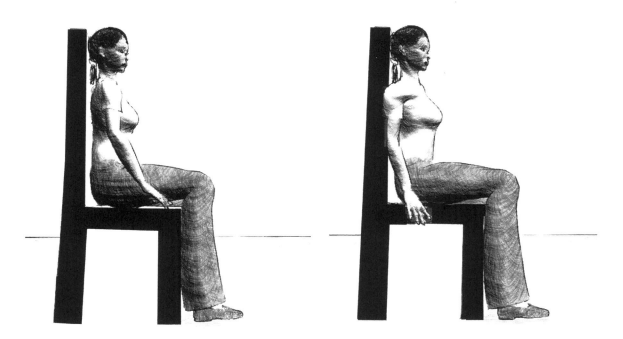

Shoulders neutral

Squeeze shoulder blades together

***Modified Shoulder Blade
Retraction***

MODIFIED SHOULDER ELEVATION/DEPRESSION

- Sit in a chair with a firm back and seat, or stand against a wall. Roll-Drop-Lock to stabilize your spine. Let your hands hang down by your sides.
- Exhale and slowly press the tops of your shoulders straight down towards the floor. Then inhale and lift the tops of your shoulders up towards your ears.
- As you do this exercise, keep your neck relaxed, head balanced, and eyes looking forward. Support your back by leaning against the wall or chair and try to feel your shoulder blades slide up and down the wall or chair.
- Repeat 5 to 10 times.
- Once you are comfortable with this movement, turn your attention to the muscles under your armpits, along the sides of your rib cage, and at the base of your shoulder blades when you exhale and lower your shoulders. Notice that it is these muscles that pull your shoulders down. Hold your shoulders down for a full breath cycle (exhale and inhale).
- Then inhale and pull your shoulders up. Hold your shoulders up by your ears for a full breath cycle (exhale and inhale) and feel the muscles in your upper back just below your neck and along the top of your shoulders engage.
- Repeat this variation 5 to 10 times.

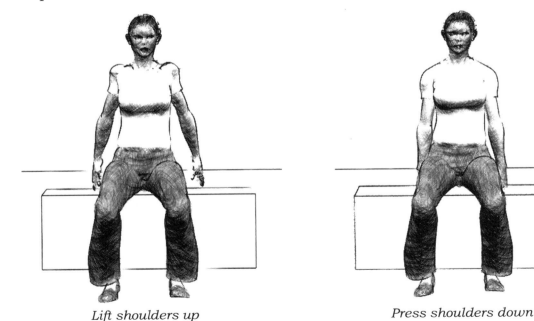

Lift shoulders up   *Press shoulders down*

Modified Shoulder Elevation/Depression

MODIFIED PULLING THE HORSE'S REIGNS

- Do not add any resistance if you have advanced osteoporosis.
- Sit toward the front of a firm seat. Roll-Drop-Lock to stabilize your spine. As you do this exercise, you should sit tall with your head balanced over your spine.
- Keep one knee bent with the foot flat on the floor. Straighten the other leg so your heel rests on the floor in front of you.
- With your palms facing each other, inhale and reach your arms forward over the extended leg. Just reach, you are not trying to touch your toes.
- Exhale, engaging your abdominals, and slide your elbows back past the lower part of your rib cage and behind you where you will squeeze your shoulder blades together.
- Relax your shoulders and neck throughout the movement. Be careful not to round your back as you reach your arms forward or arch your lower back as you squeeze your shoulder blades together.
- Repeat the movement 5 to 10 times.

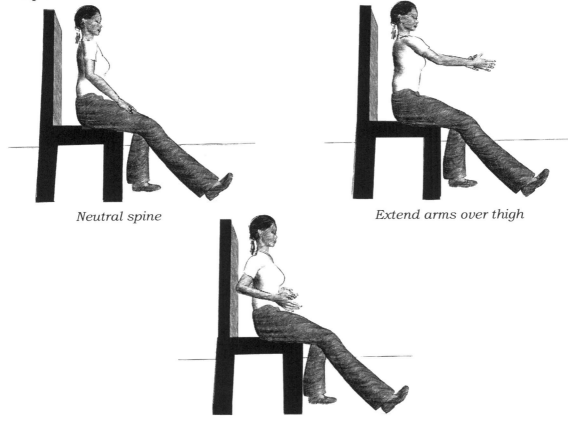

Neutral spine

Extend arms over thigh

Engage upper back

Modified Pulling The Horse's Reigns

MODIFIED UPRIGHT ROW

- Do not add resistance to these movements if you have advanced osteoporosis and be careful not to drop your chest or slouch forward. On both variations, as your elbow floats up, your shoulder should drop down towards the floor so that when your elbow is as high as you can lift it, the top of your shoulder will be as far down away from your ear as possible.
- Do this exercise while seated or standing by a sturdy table or countertop for support. You will move one arm at a time while stabilizing the other side of your body so you don't "swing your body" with the motion.
- Roll-Drop-Lock to stabilize your spine.
- First, let your arms hang down by your sides, palms facing the sides of your thighs.
- Imagine a hot air balloon is tied to one elbow and is lifting the elbow out to the side and up towards the sky. As your elbow lifts, bend it. Your hand will slide up your side towards your armpit. Keep your neck and shoulders relaxed as you lift. Then slowly lower your hand. If you feel like a gorilla scratching his armpit, you are doing it correctly!
- Repeat the movement 5 to 10 times on each arm.
- Next rotate your shoulder so your palms face the front of your thighs. Roll-Drop-Lock to stabilize your spine.
- Again, imagine a hot air balloon is tied to one elbow and is lifting it up towards the sky. As your elbow lifts, it will bend and your hand will slide up the front of your body toward your chest. Keep your neck and shoulders relaxed as you lift. Then slowly lower your hand back to your thigh.
- Repeat the movement 5 to 10 times on each arm.
- Once you can complete a full set of repetitions easily and without pain, increase your work load by lifting both elbows at the same time. When you do this, you will have to engage your core abdominal muscles even more as your elbows lift. Remember to pull your belly button in towards your spine.

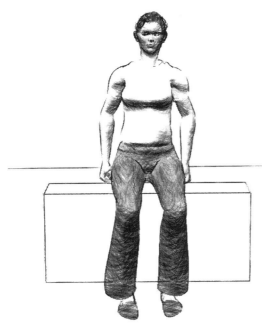

*Palms face side
of thighs*

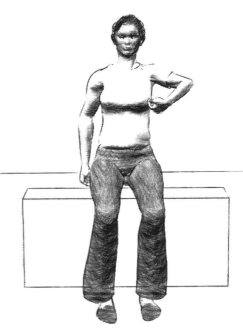

Lift palm to armpit

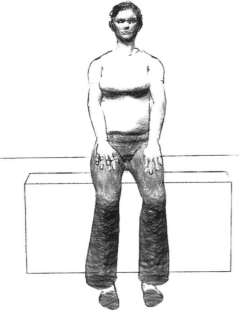

*Palms face front
of thighs*

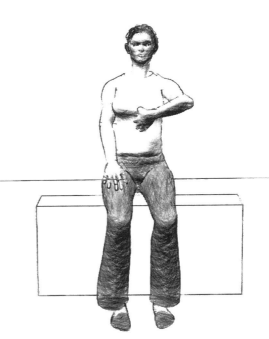

Lift palm to chest

Modified Upright Row

MODIFIED HIP AND LEG STRENGTH TRAINING FOR SEVERE OSTEOPOROSIS

The principle of counterbalance and the Rules of Engagement are especially important for you to follow if you have advanced, or severe, osteoporosis. As the exercises get more complex, the Rules of Engagement become even more important. Even though you are focusing on your lower body in these exercises, the Rules of Engagement still apply. Roll–Drop–Lock before each exercise to stabilize your shoulder girdle and pelvis. Until this stabilization becomes a habit, you may need to Roll–Drop–Lock every few repetitions.

To protect your knees, always keep your knees in line over your heels. On lunges and steps, the knee of the stepping leg should not extend forward over your toes as this puts a tremendous load on your knee joint. On the Squat, Reverse Squat, and Toe Raises, neither knee should extend forward. When you are doing the leg exercises, pause periodically to look down at your feet. If you can see your entire foot then your knee(s) are correctly aligned. If not, push your hips backward and bend your knees until you can see your entire feet. Then you know your legs are in correct alignment. Stand near a sturdy table or counter for support as you do these exercises because they will challenge your balance. As you get stronger and more confident, simply lift your hand up off the table.

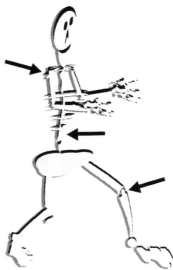

When you are doing the hip and leg exercises, focus on engaging your upper back and core muscles and keep your knee(s) aligned over your heel.

MODIFIED SQUAT AGAINST A CHAIR

- Place the back of a chair against a wall so it won't slide. If you need extra support, you can place it against a wall and next to a sturdy table or counter. Another option is to use a sturdy couch with arm rests.
- Stand in front of the chair as if you are going to sit down on it, and hold onto the table for support if needed. Scoot back until the backs of your legs touch the chair seat. This is your starting position.
- Roll-Drop-Lock to stabilize your spine. Then, without bringing the backs of your legs away from the chair, push your bottom back and allow your knees to bend around the chair seat.
- As your hips move back, your chest will come forward in counterbalance, bringing your back into a diagonal line. If you aren't holding onto a table, let your arms swing forward.
- Don't sit all the way down. Just push your hips back a few inches and feel your hips and knees bend at the same time.
- To stand upright, simply slide your hips forward so they are back in line under your shoulders. Pull your arms down next to your hips as you return to a standing position.
- Once you can do this easily for 5 to 10 repetitions, you will advance to doing the Chair Raise exercise (described next).

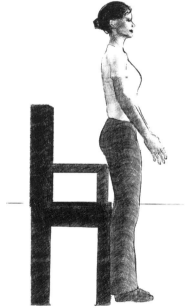

Stand with backs of legs touching chair

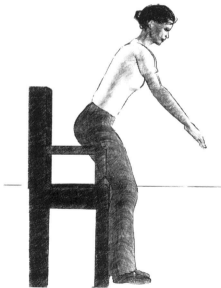

Press hips back and bring chest forward

Modified Squat Against a Chair

MODIFIED CHAIR RAISE

- Make sure you are comfortable with the Squat Against a Chair exercise before you try this exercise.
- A major goal of this exercise is to feel how physics makes movement easier. When you use the principle of counterbalance, standing up from a chair is simple.
- Sit on a firm chair with arm rests. Place your feet flat on the floor with the tops of your thighs facing up towards the ceiling and your knees hip-width apart so your toes and knees face forward. Rest your hands on the chair arms or on the seat. If you are short, you may need to scoot your bottom forward to get your feet flat on the floor. If you are unsteady, place the chair in front of a sturdy table and rest your hands on the table for support throughout the movement.
- Roll-Drop-Lock to stabilize your spine, then reach your arms out in front of your body for counterbalance.
- Keeping your belly button in and your back flat, bring your chest forward over your knees (think "nose over toes") until your bottom lifts up off the chair. At this point, push your heels into the floor, exhale and think about lifting your belly button up. Pull your arms down to your sides and slide your hips forward, straightening your body to a standing position. Your pelvis will slide forward under your chest as you move upright.
- As with a squat, keep your knees relaxed and aligned over your heels. Don't lock your knees by overextending them. Once you are standing, find your balance with equal weight over both feet.
- Return to the seat in the same manner that you did in the squat — touch the backs of your calves against the chair, push your hips back, bring your chest forward, and bend your knees around the chair seat. Slowly lower your bottom all the way down to the chair, then tilt your torso to an upright position over your pelvis. Control your body as you lower; do not just plop back down onto the chair.
- The goal is to complete this movement without pushing up off the chair with your hands, but if you need assistance, you can use your hands on the seat or table for help.
- Repeat the movement 5 to 10 times trying to make it as smooth as possible.

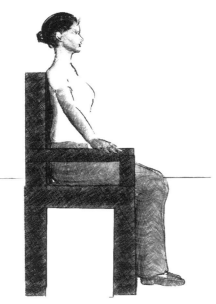

Sit upright

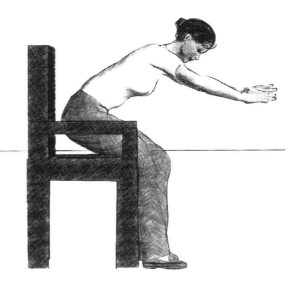

Move nose over toes

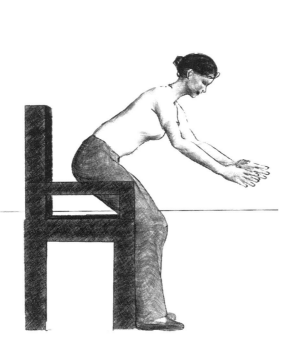

*Push heels down and
shift hips forward*

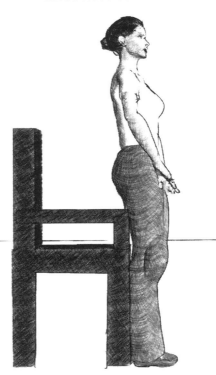

Stand upright

Modified Chair Raise

MODIFIED BACK LUNGE

- This exercise is basically a big step backward.
- Stand with your left side next to a sturdy table or counter and rest your left hand on it for support. Roll-Drop-Lock to stabilize your spine then shift your center of gravity away from the table and over your right leg.
- Lift your left knee (the one closest to the table) up in front of your body until your foot comes off the floor.
- Tilt your torso forward slightly and slowly move the lifted foot behind you. Make sure you can feel the floor behind you, then roll the balls of your toes down onto the floor. Your heel will stay up off the floor.
- Slowly shift your center of gravity back until you are equally balanced between both feet. As you shift your weight back, bend the back knee and bring it forward under your hip. Tilt your torso to an upright position. In this position both knees will be bent, your front knee will be aligned over your front heel (so you can see your entire foot), and your back heel will be off the floor.
- To step out of the lunge, make sure you are balanced, pull your belly button in toward your spine, then push off your back foot (imagine the muscles in your back leg are springs), and bring it into place next to the right one.
- Repeat 5 to 10 times stepping back onto your left leg. Then turn your body so your right side is next to the table and your right hand rests on it. Shift your center of gravity over your left leg and lunge back with your right leg 5 to 10 times.
- Keep your back straight, knees bent and focus your center of gravity so your weight is balanced between the front foot and the back foot when you are in the lunge.

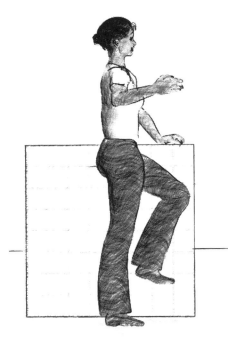

*Lift knee in front of
your body*

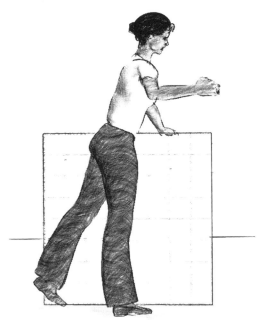

*Reach foot behind
using counterbalance*

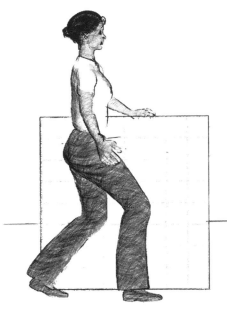

*Touch toes to floor and
shift center of gravity back*

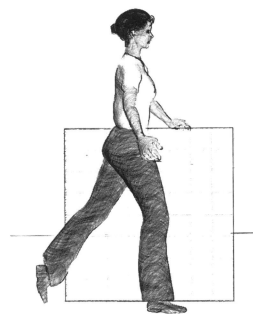

*Push off back foot and shift
center of gravity forward*

Modified Back Lunge

MODIFIED FORWARD LUNGE

- This is basically a big step forward. As with the Back Lunge, it is important to use your muscles to create the movement, not momentum, so move slowly and deliberately, bending and straightening your joints.
- Stand next to a sturdy table for assistance. With one side next to the table and your hand resting on it for support, Roll-Drop-Lock to stabilize your spine.
- Shift your center of gravity over one leg. Then bring your other knee up in front of your body to lift that foot off the floor. Extend your lifted knee and reach your the heel as far in front of you as you can.
- Bend the back knee and shift your center of gravity forward to bring the front heel down to the floor in front of you. With both knees still bent, lower your front toes down onto the floor and shift your center of gravity forward a bit more until it is centered between your feet. As you do this, your back heel will roll up off the floor. You should be in the same position as you were in the Back Lunge only the stepping foot is now forward.
- You should feel stable in this position with your front toes and heel securely on the floor, your back knee bent, and your back toes pushing down into the floor. Your back heel will stay off the floor. Check to make sure your front knee is aligned over your heel — can you see your entire front foot? If not, shift your hips backwards until you can.
- Make sure you are balanced equally between both feet. Use your muscles in the back leg as springs to push the back foot up off the floor. As your foot comes off the floor, shift your center of gravity forward, and step down into place next to the other foot.
- Continue moving forward in this manner, taking a giant step then bringing your feet together. Step forward onto one foot, spring off the back leg, and move the back leg up next to the front one. Then step forward onto the opposite foot.
- Lunge forward 4 steps then turn your body so your other side is next to the table and your other hand is your support. Roll-Drop-Lock to stabilize your spine and lunge forward alternating legs for 4 steps while stabilizing with your hand. Repeat this series until you have taken 24 steps (12 on each leg).

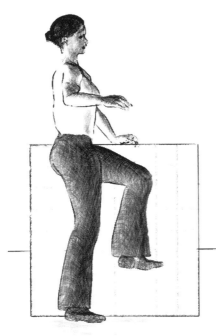

Lift knee

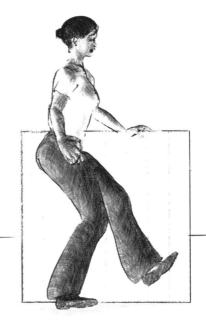

*Reach heel
forward*

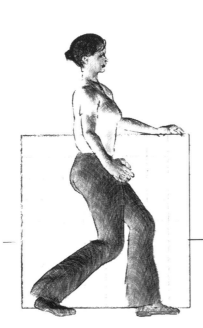

*Step down and shift
center of gravity*

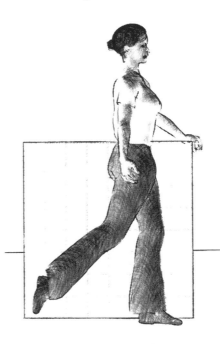

Spring off back leg

Modified Forward Lunge

MODIFIED SIDE LUNGE

- Like the other lunges, this lunge is a big step. But this time you are stepping to the side. It's amazing how many people feel uncomfortable stepping to the side, so to avoid doing it, they turn their pelvis, twist their spine, and step forward. The problem is, there are times when you must step out to the side and if you've never practiced it correctly, your muscles won't know what to do and you may injure your hip, knee, ankle, and/or back. As with the other exercises, practice using your muscles to control the movement.

- Stand facing a sturdy table or counter and rest both hands on it for support. Roll-Drop-Lock. Look at a point on the wall out in front of you. You will keep your head, pelvis, and rib cage facing that point throughout the exercise. The key to a good side lunge is to focus your mind on your center of gravity.

- Press your hips back into a mini-squat so your knees are softly bent, then shift your center of gravity over one foot. Lift the other foot off the floor, bringing that knee up in front of your body. Keep your center of gravity stable over the standing foot. Think about the outside of the ankle on your lifted foot, and slowly move it out to the side. Only move it as far to the side as you comfortably can. Practice moving your foot out to the side and back to the center a few times before continuing.

- When the lifted foot is out to the side, touch the big toe to the floor. Then, with both knees bent, push your hips back further into a squat and shift your center of gravity sideways, until it is over the foot that just touched down. As you shift your center of gravity, the rest of your toes and heel will roll down to the floor. Keep your toes and knees facing forward and your hips back to keep the stepping knee aligned over the heel.

- With your center of gravity over the new foot, lift your other foot up off the floor. Bring the lifted foot in next to the new standing leg and step down so your feet are side by side and your center of gravity is even over both feet.

- Keep your torso stable, neck relaxed, and knees aligned over your heels throughout this exercise. Focus on shifting your center of gravity from both feet, to one foot, to the other foot, and back to the center.

- Repeat 5 to 10 times on each foot.

> **Safety Note:** *It is important to move with your joints on this exercise. Don't lift your leg so high to the side that you have to tip your body to accommodate it. Lift the knee in front of you, then slide the foot to the side before you shift your weight. If you have osteoporosis in your hips, this will protect a fragile femoral neck (the section of the thigh bone that attaches to the pelvis).*

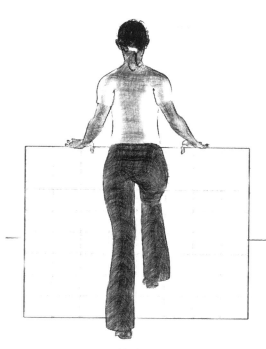

Lift knee

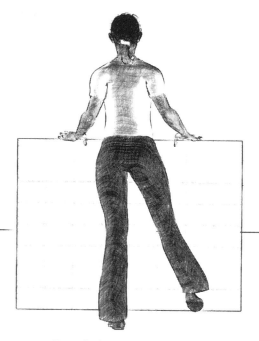

Reach foot out to the side

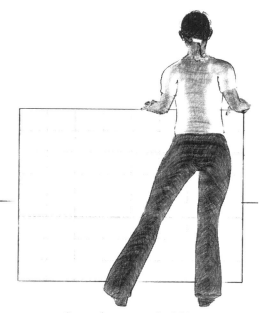

Step down and shift center of gravity

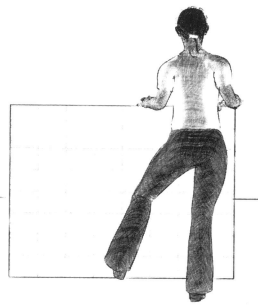

Lift opposite knee

Modified Side Lunge

MODIFIED STEPPING

- Use a handrail, wall, or chair for support and maintain good posture throughout this movement. The purpose of this step is not aerobic training but strength training. Good form is important, and the slower you move the more benefit you will obtain.
- Stand facing any step or stairway with your feet hip-width apart. Roll-Drop-Lock. Shift your center of gravity over one foot so you can lift the other foot up in front of you.
- Place your lifted foot onto the step heel first then roll the toes down onto the step. Check to make sure your entire foot is on the step. Keep your weight over the back leg so your front knee is in line over its heel.
- Imagine that your leg muscles on the back leg are springs. Coil the springs by bending the leg at the knee and lifting the heel off the floor. Now you are ready to uncoil that spring to push the back foot up off the floor and move your body up over the step. Place that foot down on the step next to the first one.
- While on the step, shift your center of gravity over one foot again and lift the other foot.
- Slowly move the lifted foot behind you and lower it to the floor. As you reach for the floor behind you, bring your chest slightly forward in counterbalance.
- When you can feel the floor under your toes, make sure both knees are bent and slowly shift your center of gravity backwards, over the back foot, in the same way you did for the Back Lunge.
- Roll the back heel down to the floor and continue to shift your center of gravity back until your belly button is aligned over the back foot.
- Then lift your front foot off of the step and bring it down to the floor next to the other one.
- Focus on the muscles in your thighs and rear end that are lifting and lowering your body.
- If necessary, look down at the step to make sure your entire foot is on the step (no toes or heels hanging off!). Never put your full weight onto the step or floor until you feel support under your foot.
- If this is too difficult, don't add it to your exercise routine until you feel stronger.
- If you can do it comfortably, repeat the movement, stepping up and down on each leg 5 to 10 times.

Step Up Heel First

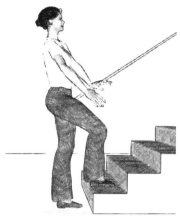

Place foot on step

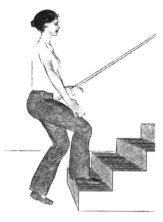

Bend back knee and lift back heel

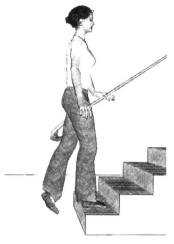

Spring up off back foot

Step Down Toes First

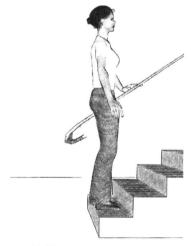

Shift center of gravity over one foot

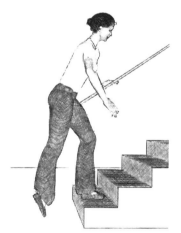

Lift opposite foot and move it behind

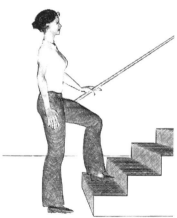

Touch floor with toes and roll down onto heel

Modified Stepping

MODIFIED TOE RAISE

- DO NOT JUMP if you have advanced osteoporosis or a current fracture. You can obtain similar benefits with this faux jump (toe raise). Always use a sturdy table or counter for support.
- Stand with your feet parallel and shoulder-width apart and your hands resting on a sturdy table or counter. Roll-Drop-Lock to stabilize your spine.
- Push your hips back a little and bend your knees, bringing your chest forward into a mini-squat position. You may feel like you are downhill skiing when in this position.
- To raise up onto your toes, slide your hips forward in the same manner you did to come out of your Squat, but this time as your body tilts upright, continue to move your center of gravity forward over your toes. Your heels will naturally lift up off the floor.
- At this point you can push up through your feet, raising your heels higher, if it feels good.
- Make sure you are balanced over the balls of your feet, including your big toes and little toes, and try to relax your toes so they spread out.
- Then allow your heels to "plop" back down to the floor bending your knees and pushing your hips behind you into a mini-squat as you land. Don't overdo the impact on your landing — you are not trying to beat your bones into submission. Your goal is to feel your balance change between a toe raise and a flat foot.
- Rise onto your toes and drop down into a mini-squat 5 to 10 times.

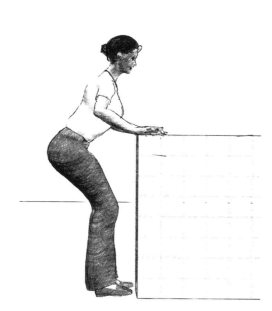

*Push hips back
into a mini-squat*

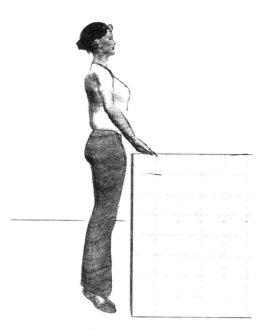

*Raise up onto
toes*

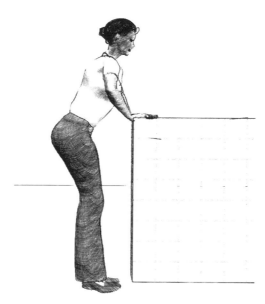

*Drop heels and
push hips back*

Modified Toe Raise

MODIFIED WRIST EXERCISES FOR SEVERE OSTEOPOROSIS

The third part of the body where we need to focus our bone-building exercise is in the wrists. Remember, the bones with the greatest percentage of trabecular bone tend to be the first ones affected by osteoporosis. The vertebra, femoral neck, and wrist are all high in trabecular bone and are the most common sites of osteoporotic fracture. These exercises will cause the muscles to tug the bones in your wrists in all directions, ultimately increasing bone strength. They will improve your range of motion as well.

All of these exercises can be done from either a seated or standing position. These exercises may cause pain if you've had a fracture in your wrist or have arthritis in your wrist, fingers, or hand. Don't try to do this if a fracture hasn't yet healed. If it hurts, try making the movement smaller or rotating your hand to a different position. If these modifications don't relieve your pain, then don't do the exercise. Work towards a greater range of motion slowly and gently.

MODIFIED WRIST CIRCLES

- You can do this exercise while sitting or standing. Roll-Drop-Lock to stabilize your spine.
- Grip a pencil in your fingers as if you are going to write and imagine you are sitting or standing in front of a big, blank wall.
- Let your elbows drop down next to your rib cage.
- Holding the pencil in front of your chest, draw a circle on that wall by moving your wrist in a circle. Be careful, your elbow and shoulder will try to do the motion for your wrist. Stabilize your elbow and shoulder by bringing your elbow in against the side of your rib cage. You can also stabilize the arm by holding onto your elbow or forearm with the other hand.
- Watch the shape your hand draws and strive for a precise, smooth, round circle. Draw circles in one direction then in the other. As you get good at drawing circles, add figure 8's and alphabet letters.
- Repeat the movement 5 to 10 times using each hand.

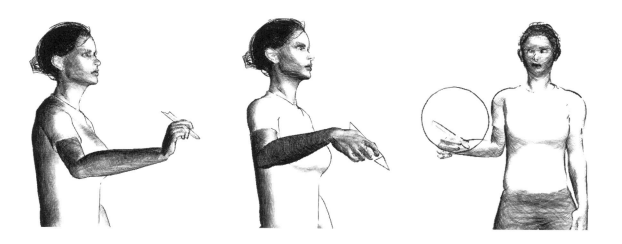

Modified Wrist Circles

MODIFIED WRIST HYPEREXTENSION

- Sit or stand with your feet parallel and a little wider than hip-width apart. Roll-Drop-Lock and let your arms hang down in front of your body, palms facing your thighs.
- **Press Forward:** Bend your elbows to bring your hands up to chest height, palms facing the floor. When your hands reach chest height, turn your fingertips up toward the ceiling.
  - With your palms facing away from your body, press the base of your palms straight out in front of your chest, straightening your elbows. Try to hold your arms up at shoulder height with your wrists bent back and your fingertips pointed up as if you were pushing against a wall in front of you. However, if you need to keep your arms lower that is fine. Focus on pressing the base of your palms away from your body to get full hyperextension of the wrists.
  - Then relax your wrists allowing your palms to face the floor. Without tightening your neck or the tops of your shoulders, slide your elbows back along your sides to bring your hands back towards your chest.
- **Press To The Sides:** Next, from the position in front of your chest, pull your fingertips up again and rotate your shoulders outward so your palms face to the side.
  - Imagine you are in a narrow hallway and push your palms outward as if you are pushing the base of your palms against the walls beside you.
  - Relax your wrists and bring your elbows back in beside your rib cage.
- **Press Down:** Relax your arms and let them hang down beside your thighs with your palms rotated to face behind you.
  - Lift your elbows up behind you so your hands rest next to your waist. Your palms will still be facing behind you.
  - Pull your fingertips back, so your wrist is in hyperextension and your palms face the floor. Press the base of your palms down toward the floor as if you were pressing on a table, straightening your elbows.
  - Relax your wrists and let your arms hang by your sides.
- Repeat the three motions (pressing to the front, to the sides, and down) 5 to 10 times.
- To help keep your neck and the tops of your shoulders relaxed, imagine that your hands are the wings of a butterfly, gently fluttering with the movement of your arms. Because this motion requires you to engage your upper back muscles, you must follow the Rules of Engagement.
- If you experience any pain in your neck, shoulders, or back as you do these exercises, move one hand at a time while resting the other hand down by your side.

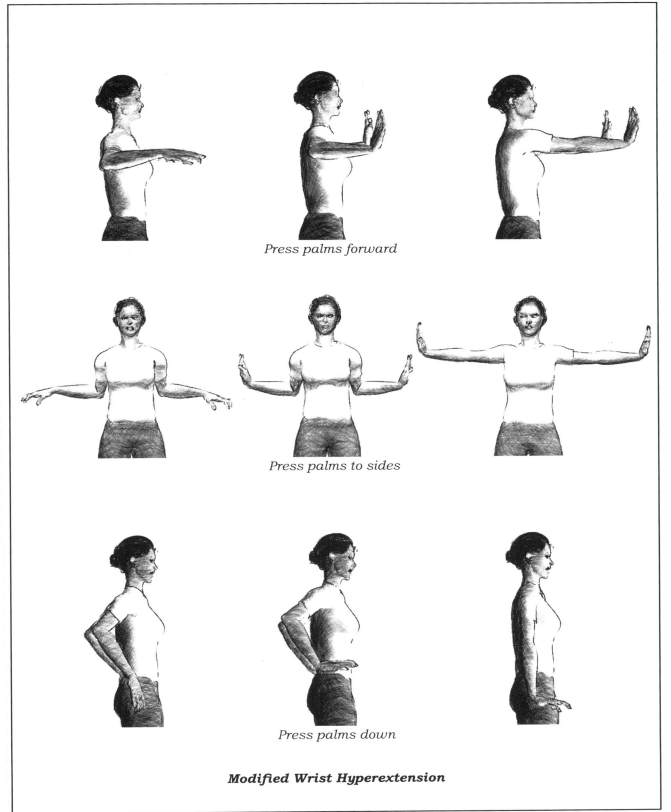

Press palms forward

Press palms to sides

Press palms down

Modified Wrist Hyperextension

MODIFIED PLAY THE PIANO

- While sitting or standing, let your arms hang in front of your body, palms facing your thighs.
- Bend your elbows to bring your hands up in front of your tummy, palms down as if your fingers are resting on piano keys. Keep your torso stable and shoulders relaxed. If this position causes discomfort in your neck or shoulders, rest your hands on a tabletop, palms down.
- Turn your wrists out to the sides – turning both wrists outward at the same time. As you move your wrists outward, your goal is to bring the pinkies closer to the outside of your forearm.
- Then turn both wrists inward. When you bring your wrists inward, bring the thumbs closer to the inside of your forearms.
- It is important to keep your wrists lifted and your fingers resting on the imaginary piano keys. Keep this movement in your wrists, don't allow your shoulders to move. If you need to, you can hold one forearm with your other hand and move one wrist at a time.
- Repeat in both directions 5 to 10 times.

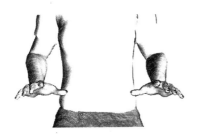
Wrists neutral

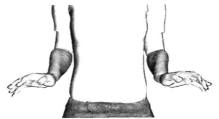
Wrists turn out

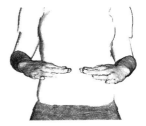
Wrists turn in

Modified Play The Piano

8

Supplements and Medications

The information provided here regarding supplements and medications is intended solely for general information and should not be relied upon for any particular diagnosis, treatment, or care. Medication options change often so your decision to use, or not use, any medication should come after a thorough discussion with your physician and a careful analysis of your risk factors and osteoporosis tests. Likewise, as research uncovers a greater understanding of how different nutrients contribute to bone health, updates will be made concerning vitamin and mineral supplementation. Inclusion in this list does not imply an endorsement of any particular medication or manufacturer by the author, publisher, or any of the references cited. For detailed information on the actions, administration and possible side effects for each of the following medications, please consult the package inserts, available on-line and at pharmacies.

Vitamin and Mineral Supplements

In some cases, the B O N and E of your BONES Lifestyle won't be enough to ward off osteoporosis. If you have numerous risk factors or haven't gotten results with the other elements of the lifestyle, you may need to include the S of the BONES Lifestyle, supplementation and/or medication.

Vitamin and mineral supplementation may help boost your bone-building cycle up to an acceptable rate of bone regeneration. The benefits of nutrients are greatest when they are obtained through food. But good nutrition is only as good as the absorption of the nutrients you eat. If you have an illness that affects your body's absorption of nutrients or there are certain foods you cannot eat, you could be at a higher risk for osteoporosis.

You and your physician may determine that it is necessary to add supplements to your diet. Calcium and Vitamin D are essential for bone health and often require supplementation, but you may also need to supplement other vitamins and minerals as well.

Confirm that you are either eating or supplementing enough of each bone-healthy vitamin and mineral. The recommended daily allowance varies from person to person, so it is best to work with your physician and a registered dietician to determine your dosage requirements for each vitamin and mineral.

> *In one study researchers discovered that 50% of the women in their study who were hospitalized for hip fractures were deficient in vitamin D.*

Bone-Healthy Vitamins and Minerals That May Require Supplementation

Vitamins	Minerals
Vitamin A	Calcium
Vitamin B5	Magnesium
Vitamin B6	Phosphorus
Vitamin B9	Potassium
Vitamin B12	Boron
Vitamin C	Copper
Vitamin D	Manganese
Vitamin E	Silica
Vitamin K	Sulfur
	Zinc

HOW TO

KNOW IF YOU SHOULD TAKE VITAMIN/MINERAL SUPPLEMENTS

In most cases, it is safe to add a daily supplement to provide necessary nutrients that you may be missing. Just be aware that when you add vitamin/mineral supplements, too much of a good thing can negate the benefits and may even be harmful. Doctors like to use the phrase, "the dose makes the poison."

For example, too much vitamin A can actually increase your risk of bone fracture. It appears that excessive amounts of vitamin A (above 10,000 IU) triggers an increase in the work of the bone crushers (osteoclasts). In addition, too much vitamin A may interfere with vitamin D absorption. Vitamin A in the form of beta carotene doesn't seem to be as dangerous as vitamin A in the form of retinol. If you are getting your vitamin A through food sources, you are probably fine. If you take supplements that contain this vitamin, be sure to check your total intake. Some supplements contain more than four times the recommended dietary allowance of vitamin A.

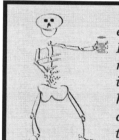

Some supplements don't easily dissolve in your stomach. How can you tell if your supplement is easily digestible? Drop it into a glass of vinegar and wait half an hour. If it is completely dissolved after that half hour, then it's digestible.

Calcium can also cause problems. Supplemental calcium is available in many different forms. Which form is the best one? In general, you want a form of calcium that is soluble (meaning that it will dissolve in your stomach). The words that follow calcium on your nutrition label are the chemicals that bind with the calcium to make it stable. The cheapest, most common supplement is calcium carbonate. Tums® antacids are made of calcium carbonate. But because Tums® is an antacid, it reduces your stomach acidity and may actually decrease absorption of the calcium. Furthermore, by binding with other minerals and vitamins, it may limit their absorption as well. Since calcium can only be absorbed 500mg at a time and is best absorbed when taken with food, the type of calcium you take and the time of day that you take it are both important.

The main number you want to know when selecting a calcium supplement is the amount of elemental calcium it provides. The problem is that not all labels will tell you this amount.

In general, the amount of elemental calcium in the different forms is as follows:
- Calcium carbonate = 40% elemental calcium provided
- Calcium citrate = 21% elemental calcium provided
- Calcium lactate = 13% elemental calcium provided
- Calcium gluconate = 9% elemental calcium provided

It seems logical to add supplements to your diet if they may help you prevent an illness, but be careful. We often run into trouble when we try to mix and match to create our own multivitamins. Remember, you learned in Chapter 6 that there are at least 22 known vitamins and minerals that your bones need. Instead of trying to build your own vitamin/mineral portfolio, a better approach would be to add a multivitamin that contains all of the necessary nutrients in a prescribed dosage. Show your doctor your multivitamin to make certain it is right for your needs. Ask if you should add a secondary calcium/vitamin D supplement.

If you are going to take a vitamin or mineral supplement, read the label carefully and follow any instructions on it. If you are uncertain about the safety of a nutritional supplement or have questions about it, check with your health care provider before taking it. If you aren't sure what supplements to add, a registered dietitian or nutritionist can be very helpful.

Medication

Often, supplementation alone will not be enough to stave off osteoporosis. In this case, your doctor may also recommend medication.

Most of the drugs prescribed today for osteoporosis are **antiresorptive**, which means they stop the resorption (breakdown) of old bone. Bisphosphonates, calcitonin, and estrogen or hormone replacement therapies (ERT or HRT), are all antiresorptive drugs. They work by suppressing the bone remodeling system. By inhibiting the bone crushers (osteoclasts), they slow down bone removal and the release of minerals into the blood. Since these drugs do not affect the bone builders (osteoblasts), new bone formation continues and, in theory, overall bone density and bone strength increases.

The problem is, remodeling is the body's way of preventing and repairing damage to the bone. So when these drugs suppress the remodeling process, fatigue damage can occur and reduce the bone's ability to absorb energy. This could lead to fatigue fractures.

Formative drugs that stimulate the osteoblasts and encourage new bone growth are few. Currently, there are only two available — teriparatide and sodium fluoride. Teriparatide is a newly approved drug for severe osteoporosis. It is a parathyroid hormone that builds bone by stimulating osteoblasts to form new bone. Sodium flouride has not yet been approved by the FDA to treat osteoporosis. Although some of the data shows promising results with this treatment, other studies suggest that the new bone formed is more brittle and susceptible to fractures. This is probably because, while flouride affects the size and shape of the bone crystals, it doesn't encourage corresponding changes in the collagen fibers that give bone its flexibility. This treatment shows promise but requires further research and development.

In the past, ERT or HRT was commonly prescribed. Because of potentially serious side effects, including an increased risk of cardiovascular disease, stroke, breast cancer, and gallbladder disease, estrogen and hormone therapy are no longer recommended for treatment of osteoporosis. Also, while effective at reducing bone loss and increasing bone mineral density in the spine and hip as long as it is being taken, once discontinued, bone loss returns to its normal course. So you are just putting off the inevitable with ERT and HRT.

Bisphosphonates are currently the first choice of osteoporosis treatment for most physicians. New synthetic hormones called selective estrogen receptor modulators (SERMS) are sometimes used instead of bisphosphonates and another drug now being prescribed is a hormone called calcitonin. This hormone is involved in calcium regulation and bone metabolism. It has been shown to slow bone loss and increase bone density in the spine. It may also relieve the pain associated with bone fractures in women who are more than 5 years postmenopausal.

HOW TO

KNOW IF YOU SHOULD YOU TAKE MEDICATION

The choice to take medication to prevent or treat osteoporosis is a personal decision. It should be based on your risk factors for osteoporosis and other diseases such as cancer or heart disease. If you have already suffered a fracture due to bone loss then the answer would likely be yes. If not, the best indicator would be multiple DEXA scans showing a clear decrease in your bone mineral density over time combined with lab tests that show an increased excretion of urinary collagen and calcium. Ideally, you will combine any drug therapy with exercise, good nutrition, and supplementation. Many studies show that a combination of these treatments yields the best overall results. Exercise, in particular, helps the medication provide the greatest benefit.

Available research recommends the least intrusive action possible. If you have only had one bone scan, and it shows low bone mineral density in comparison to other women aged 25-35, you are a good candidate for an osteoporosis exercise and nutrition program. Vitamin supplements will provide additional nutrients that are probably missing from your diet. If after a 2nd or 3rd test your bone density is shown to be decreasing, then consider adding medication. Work with your doctor to identify all your risk factors and determine appropriate lifestyle changes.

Treating osteoporosis with medication has been most effective for women with multiple risk factors and T-scores of less than –2.5. The benefits of medication are not as significant for men, or for women with T-scores above – 2.5. The effects of drug treatment on men and women with osteopenia are not yet clear. By ordering necessary tests, your doctor can help you assess your situation so you can make the best choice.

All medications have potential side effects. Before you start taking any medicine, be sure you understand what these are and how they may affect you. In some cases, the side effects will outweigh the benefits and you may not want to take the medication. The most common side effects of osteoporosis medications include gastrointestinal disturbances, pain, or allergic reactions. Some, such as estrogen and hormone replacement therapies, have serious risks — cardiovascular disease, stroke, blood clots, or breast cancer. Be sure to talk to your doctor about the risks and benefits of taking medication for osteoporosis so you are confident that the medicine prescribed is right for you.

The following chart shows the pros, cons, and possible side effects of osteoporosis medications.

Formative Drugs That Stimulate Bone Formation

Drug	Pros	Cons	Possible Side effects	Usage
Teriparatide (Brand name Forteo®)	• Parathyroid hormone that stimulates osteoblasts and forms new bone faster than old bone is broken down • Increases bone mineral density in the spine to a much greater degree in a shorter period of time than bisphosphonates	• Increases calcium absorption, so daily calcium supplements should not exceed 1000 mg and total calcium intake from all sources should not exceed 1500 mg daily • Expensive	• Only approved for a lifetime exposure of 18 months • Dizziness, nausea, or leg cramps • Hypercalcemia (increased calcium) may rarely occur • Increased risk of bone cancer in rats	• For cases of severe osteoporosis • Taken as a daily injection • Approved for use by both men and women • Not recommended for people with severe kidney impairment, primary hyperparathyroidism, hypercalcemia, or Paget's disease • Not recommended for pregnant women, children, or adolescents • Not for use by anyone with a history of radiation therapy involving the skeleton or with bone metastases
Sodium Flouride	• Activates osteoblasts (bone builders) • Increases size and shape of bone mineral crystals	• New bone may be brittle		• Not yet approved for treatment of osteoporosis

Antiresorptive Drugs That Inhibit Bone Breakdown

Drug	Pros	Cons	Possible Side Effects	Usage
Bisphospho-nates *Alendronate (brand name, Fosamax®)* *Ibandronate (brand name Boniva®)* *Risedronate (brand name Actonel®)*	• Slow down osteoclasts (bone crushers) • Remain in the bone for years so may remain effective even after usage has stopped • Alendronate and Rise-dronate may be taken daily or weekly • Ibandronate is taken once a month. Binds with bones so it continues to work throughout the month	• Must be taken on an empty stomach first thing in the morning, at least 30 to 60 minutes before eating or drinking and you must remain upright during this 30 to 60-minute period • Must take 1500mg of Calcium and 400 to 800 IU of vitamin D daily with this medication • Must take this medicine with water because water doesn't affect the drug's absorption in the stomach	• Gastrointestinal problems, abdominal pain, nausea, heartburn, or irritation of the esophagus • Bone, joint, and/or muscle pain. Stopping use of the medication typically stops the pain • Osteonecrosis of the jaw (severe infection and rotting in the jaw that leads to the death of bone tissue) • Atypical femoral fracture • Eye inflammation	• First choice of drugs for many physicians • Alendronate and Rise-dronate are approved for use by both men and women • Ibandronate is approved for use only in women • Do not take if you have acid reflux disease, esophageal strictures, kidney disease, or vitamin D deficiency
Estrogen and Hormone Replacement (ERT and HRT)	• Reduces frequency of the bone remodeling cycle • Decreases activity of osteoclasts (bone crushers) • Increases collagen production • Stimulates activation of vitamin D	• Does not repair or replace bone that has been lost • Once discontinued, bone loss accelerates to nontreatment levels	• Cardiovascular disease, stroke, blood clots, breast cancer or endometrial cancer • Vaginal bleeding, breast tenderness, headaches and depression	• No longer recommended due to potentially serious side effects • Approved only for women

Drug	Pros	Cons	Possible Side Effects	Usage
Selective Estrogen Receptor Modulators (SERMS) *Raloxifene (Brand name Evista®)*	• Synthetic hormones that have been developed to provide the beneficial effects of estrogen replacement therapy without the potential risks • Take daily with or without meals • Reduces the risk of spinal fractures	• No proof that it can reduce the risk of hip and other non-spinal fractures	• Hot flashes, sweating, flu-like symptoms, joint pain, muscle spasm, leg cramps • Swelling, water retention in the legs • Headaches, weight gain, infections, insomnia, or depression • Increased risk of blood clots, stroke, loss of vision, gallstones, or uterine bleeding • Allergic reactions	• For women only • Do not take if you are nursing, pregnant, or may become pregnant • Not recommended for people with kidney or liver problems • Do not take Raloxifene along with estrogen in the form of pills, patches, or injections
Other Hormones *Calcitonin (Brand name Miacalcin®, Calcimar® or Fortical®)*	• Hormone involved in bone metabolism and calcium regulation • Slows bone loss • Increases spinal bone density • May relieve pain associated with bone fractures	• No evidence to show a decreased risk of non-spinal fractures	• Possible allergic reaction • Flushing of the face and hands, urinary frequency, nausea, skin rash, nasal irritation, backache, bloody nose, or headaches • Some women may develop resistance to the drug after prolonged use	• For women who are more than 5 years beyond menopause • Taken as an injection or nasal spray • Approved only for use by women

9

On The Horizon

Tissue Regeneration

One of the most exciting new technologies being developed is tissue regeneration. Like a salamander, humans apparently have the ability to re-grow injured body parts. While still in the womb, fetuses can regenerate tissue that gets damaged, but this ability seems to shut off once the fetus is fully developed. Regenerative medicine is actively researching the potential of the human body to re-grow body parts — even entire limbs. Early results are promising, showing re-growth in a similar manner to the way that deer re-grow lost antlers, which are made up of cartilage, bone, tissue, and skin.

At the University of Pittsburgh, Dr. Stephen Badylak is experimenting with a powder called extracellular matrix. This powder is made up of mostly collagen that is extracted from pig's bladder. When applied, it directs the cells to divide, differentiate, and organize themselves into a specific form. In other words, this powder, sometimes called 'pixie dust,' lays a down a blueprint that the cells use to rebuild tissue. The hope is that scientists can learn how to trigger the human extracellular matrix to start working again.

In one publicized case, a hobby store owner sliced off the tip of his finger down to the top of the bone. Instead of accepting a shortened finger with a skin graft, he chose to try the extracellular matrix powder. He applied it to the fingertip and

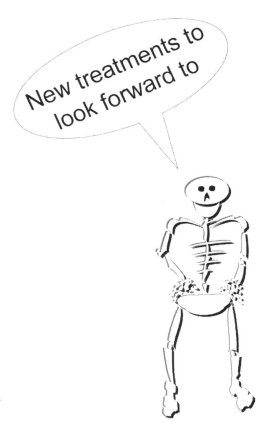

New treatments to look forward to

a few months later, he had completely re-grown the finger — skin, tissue, nerves, and fingernail included. Veterinarians are currently using it to repair horses' torn ligaments and doctors are looking for new ways to utilize the 'magic' pixie dust.

At this time, the extracellular matrix has not been able to regrow bone, but research is underway on military personnel who have injured their hands during the Iraq War. Dr. Badylak is enthusiastic about this treatment option. "I think that within ten years we will have strategies that will re-grow the bones and promote the growth of functional tissue around those bones."

Site-Directed Bone Growth (SDBG)

Research into another form of tissue regeneration is also underway. Site-Directed Bone Growth, or SDBG, is a method of encouraging bone formation by culturing osteoblasts (bone builders) on a bone's surface. Results of early-stage studies done by researchers at Yale University School of Medicine and the company Unigene have shown that with SDBG, the newly formed bone tissue on rats appears to be structurally and biologically normal and demonstrates improved biomechanical properties. Additional studies that extend the results of this work in different animal models are ongoing.

Plans for treatment with this method involve the use of an outpatient procedure combined with administration of an anabolic drug to facilitate and accelerate natural bone growth at precisely targeted locations. Researchers suggest that possible applications of this technology include strengthening bones weakened by osteoporosis, repairing damaged or fractured bones, treating chronic back pain, preventing hip fractures, and improving bone healing. "This technology could radically change the way patients are currently treated for weakened or fractured hips, vertebrae and acute traumatic long bone fractures," stated Dr. Agnès Vignery, principal investigator at Yale

University and senior author of the publication. "Physicians currently treat such conditions using invasive techniques that require operating room time, utilize artificial materials, and result in imperfect outcomes. The ideal approach would be to create new bone where it is needed and at a faster rate." According to Vignery, "Most drugs affect the whole body. But our treatment increases bone density just where it's needed."

There is no clear time line as to when this therapy might be available to people with osteoporosis, but it's definitely something to keep an eye on.

Vibration Therapy

NASA has funded studies to discover new ways to prevent bone loss in astronauts when they are in space for prolonged periods of time. One solution that is in the works is to have astronauts stand on a lightly vibrating plate for 10 to 20 minutes each day. As you learned in earlier chapters, bone cells seem to create an electrical impulse that stimulates new bone growth. You also learned how exercise appears to create a similar impulse. Recent research suggests that vibration therapy encourages an electrical stimulus within the bone.

The theory is that along with significant stresses that signal bone to form, there are also small, high frequency vibrations that occur with daily use of muscles that signal the bone remodeling system. The vibrations used in this therapy mimic the small, high frequency ones created by regular muscle contractions. If it is true that these small, regular stimuli have a big impact on bone remodeling, then a short period of time spent each day on a vibrating plate may provide the necessary signals to maintain bone strength.

The vibrations used in this type of therapy are subtle, but preliminary studies have shown a positive effect on bone. To study the effects of vibration therapy, the astronauts strapped themselves to a vibrating plate with a belt and worked on other tasks while they vibrated. It appears to counter the effects of weightlessness and prevent bone loss in the astronauts.

In studies done on animals, vibration therapy caused an increase in trabecular bone strength of 25% and doubled the rate of bone formation. Furthermore, treatment appears to enhance muscle strength and improve postural stability and balance which will improve functional strength and help prevent fractures. The hope is that this therapy may one day be useful for treating and preventing osteoporosis and osteoporosis-related fractures.

The effects of such therapy are not completely known for people who are susceptible to osteoporosis. In research done at the State University of New York, it was found that vibration therapy may have the potential to prevent bone loss in postmenopausal women, with the greatest benefit occurring in the spines of lighter women with low body mass indexes. But the level and length of vibrations used in the study failed to form new bone. Variables such as age, nutrition, exercise habits, genetic makeup, compliance, and socio-economic factors must also be considered before conclusions can be made as to the effectiveness of vibration therapy in treating osteoporosis.

Beware of commercial machines that claim to enhance athletic performance with vibration therapy. They may actually damage bone and soft tissue with vibrations that are too strong. It has not yet been determined how much vibration is safe and effective for treating weak bones. But with the positive results of these early studies, more research is underway and the effectiveness of this treatment for the general population should soon become clear.

Electrical or Ultrasound Bone Growth Stimulation

For many years, scientists have been measuring the effects of electrical current on bone growth. The idea is that a low electrical current will stimulate the bone remodeling cycle and speed the healing of bone fractures. It also appears that specific frequencies are able to inhibit bone loss. So far, results are positive for helping slow-healing bones mend. When used to treat a fracture, electromagnetic coils are placed on either side of a fracture and a pulsating electromagnetic field passes through the bone.

At this time, electromagnetic stimulation is used to help difficult fractures heal, but some experts believe it may be beneficial for rebuilding bone loss due to osteoporosis and for preventing future bone loss. It is prohibitive for many people because it is time consuming and expensive. It must be done for three to ten hours per day for at least three to six months to be effective.

A newer treatment option for stimulating bone growth is ultrasound. In this therapy, low intensity sound waves are massaged over the skin around the fracture site for about 20 to 30 minutes per day. It is thought that this will stimulate bone growth in much the same way as an electrical current does. However, not a lot of research has been done in this area yet.

Success in both of these areas depends on the severity of the fracture as well as the location and type of fracture. The overall health, age, and compliance of the patient also make a difference as to the effectiveness.

Genes That Contribute to Osteoporosis

Before long, you may be able to predict your chance of developing osteoporosis with a simple genetic test. Genetic scientists have discovered that certain versions of the BMP-2 gene may account for an increased risk of developing osteoporosis. If you have one of these versions, it does not guarantee you will develop osteoporosis, but it may increase your risk up to 3 times. It is estimated that about 10% of the population has one of them.

As research teams work to develop tests to identify people who have these genes, they can also develop better medications for osteoporosis based on their findings. People with one of the genes can also start a focused BONES Lifestyle as early as possible to prevent the devastating side-effects of osteoporosis.

10

Living The BONES Lifestyle©

The bone you build in your youth is a major determinant of your osteoporosis risk later in life. If you build up a good base throughout your childhood, you will step into adulthood with stronger bones and a larger mineral account to draw from later in life. Once your peak bone mineral density has been reached at about age 25, you cannot add additional bone density. You can only replace what has been lost due to aging, lifestyle, medications, and illnesses. This doesn't mean you can't increase your bone mineral density if a bone mineral density scan shows you have lost bone. With proper care, it is possible to bring it back to the peak level you had in your late 20s.

The cause of osteoporosis is not yet fully understood but it is apparent that bone loss is due to a variety of factors, each one building on the others. These bone-depleting factors add up until the total load is more than the bones can handle. Although many risk factors for bone loss such as age, genetics, illness, and gender are out of your control, about 50% of the risk factors for osteoporosis are lifestyle-related.

It's never too late to start practicing a BONES Lifestyle. Make the effort to develop new, positive habits. Good nutrition, regular exercise, and avoidance of bone robbers will go a long way toward preventing osteoporosis. There are also some simple habits you can develop that will help prevent bone damage.

> *Exercise and a balanced diet both positively affect collagen content and osteoblast activity (bone building) and deter osteoclast activity (bone crushing). Most current medications just deter osteoclast activity – bone crushing.*

HOW TO

PROTECT YOUR BONES DURING DAILY ACTIVITIES

It's safer to push than to pull

Pulling creates excess strain on the vertebrae. If you must move a heavy object, keep your knees slightly bent, Roll-Drop-Lock to stabilize your spine and engage your core abdominals, then push the item. You can push from either a squat position with your feet side-by-side and wider than shoulder-width or from a lunge position with one foot in front of the other. Place the object on wheels or sliders if at all possible.

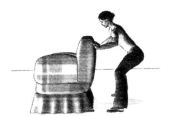 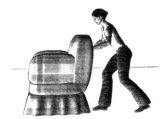

When picking up an object, use a squat position

Stand over the object you plan to lift. Place your feet parallel to each other, straddling the object. Roll-Drop-Lock to keep your spine in a neutral position. Push your hips back and bring your chest forward into a squat over the object. As with the Squat exercise in Chapter 7, bend your knees as your hips go back. Look down to be sure you can see your entire feet. Continue to push your hips back and down until you can grasp the object. Engage your core abdominals by pulling your belly button in toward your spine. Exhale and pull your elbows back to lift the object up to your body. Try to bring the object directly in toward your center of gravity (just below your belly button). Then push your heels into the floor and slide your pelvis and center of gravity forward to stand up straight. Carry the item close to your center of gravity, using both hands, with elbows bent, and your upper back and abdominal muscles engaged. If you feel strain in your lower back while carrying, pull your bellybutton in and bend your knees a bit more as you walk.

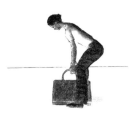 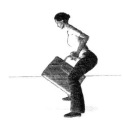 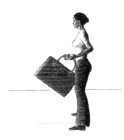

When lifting or carrying items, the closer you hold them to your center of gravity, the better

As your load moves away from your center of gravity, the weight increases exponentially. Carry items close to your center of gravity and split heavy loads into separate lighter ones if possible.

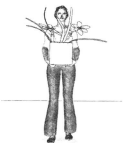

When carrying multiple items, plan ahead

Heavy loads place excessive strain on the vertebrae and make you less balanced. Carry groceries or suitcases evenly balanced between both sides or push them in front of you on a wheeled cart. Separate heavy loads into multiple lighter ones and make more trips.

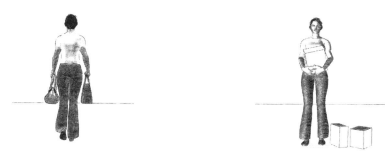

Avoid movements that twist and bend your spine at the same time

This applies when you are sitting or standing. Don't reach to the floor beside your chair to pick something up or to the back seat of your car to grab something. This is a common cause of back strain and could fracture a weak vertebra. Instead, place needed objects in front of you or up at hand height beside you for easy access, move your feet and turn your whole body, or stand over the object and squat down to retrieve it.

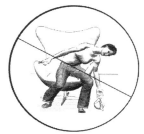
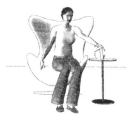

When pushing a shopping cart, walker, or wheelchair, stand upright and move the cart forward with your legs, not your back

If the handles are adjustable, set them high enough so you can stand upright when you hold them. To maintain good shoulder alignment, keep your hands relaxed on the handles. Roll-Drop-Lock and bring your elbows in close to your rib cage to lock your arms and torso. This way, you will move the cart forward with your legs pushing your torso. Bend one knee, lifting the foot off the floor. Straighten that knee bringing your foot closer to the cart, touch the heel to the floor, then push off the back foot to shift your center of gravity forward over the front foot and roll down onto your toes. Do not bend forward or round your back while you push the cart as this will strain your vertebrae. If you pull your belly button in and let the cart roll as your back leg pushes forward, you shouldn't hit the cart with your knee.

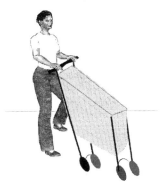

To maintain correct spinal alignment when you sleep, add extra pillows

If you sleep on your side, place a pillow between your knees and another pillow supporting your upper arm. If you sleep on your back, put a pillow under your knees. Use a pillow under your head that supports and maintains the natural curve of your neck. You don't want your neck to be placed at a sharp angle. Avoid sleeping on your stomach because it places too much strain on your neck and lower back.

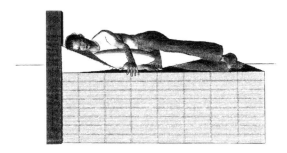

When getting out of or into bed, roll smoothly onto your side first then bring your feet off or on the bed

To get out of bed, exhale to engage your core and roll onto your side, turning your pelvis and rib cage together as a unit. Place your lower elbow on the bed for support, and bring your feet off the edge of the bed. Use both arms to help shift your weight over both hips so you are in a seated position. Lower your feet to the floor while still sitting. If your feet don't reach the floor, slide one foot down to the floor at a time while leaning against the bed. Feel the weight over your heels, push your hips back slightly and bring your chest forward (think "nose over toes") until your bottom lifts off the bed. Once your hips are off the bed, keep your weight evenly distributed over both feet. Push your heels into the floor and pull your hips forward in line over your feet. As your hips come forward, let your chest tilt upright to line up over your hips.

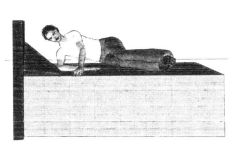 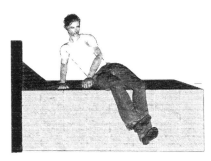

To get into bed, stand next to the bed, with the backs of both legs touching the bed. Press your hips back and bring your chest forward into a squat. Then slowly lower your bottom onto the bed, resting your hands on the bed, night stand, or a cane as you lower. Once you are sitting on the bed, lower the shoulder that is next to your pillow down onto the bed, and roll your feet up onto the bed. To roll over, engage your core and move your rib cage and pelvis at the same time so you don't over rotate your spine.

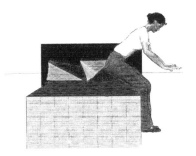 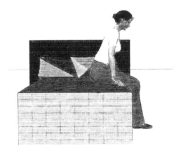

When gardening or playing with children or pets, lower yourself into a lunge position then set one knee down on the ground or onto a pad

While you are on one knee, keep the other foot flat on the floor and your back straight. Make sure you are engaging your core abdominals. It's best to kneel on a pad or pillow. If this hurts your knee, sit tall on a step stool or chair.

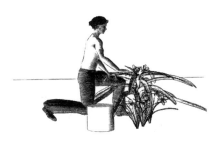

When washing dishes or brushing your teeth at the sink, roll-drop-lock to stabilize your spine and change position by moving your hips and knees.

Stand with your feet side-by-side. Keep your weight evenly balanced over both feet and your rear end and knees relaxed. Roll-Drop-Lock to stabilize your spine. To bend over the sink, press your hips back into a squat and bend your knees, bringing your chest and head forward with a flat back. If you experience back pain when standing at a counter or sink, try resting one foot on a step stool. Change positions and take frequent breaks to prevent your back muscles from overworking. Don't allow yourself to slouch or round your back.

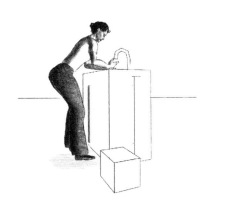 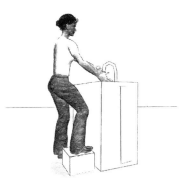

To get up from the ground, use a lunge position

Kneel on one knee and bend the ankle so the balls of that foot's toes are on the floor. Place the other foot in front of you with the foot flat on the floor and the knee directly over the heel. Roll-Drop-Lock, push your front heel down into the floor, and press your hands down on the thigh of the front leg. If you prefer, you can press your hands down on the seat of a chair next to you. Straighten the back leg to bring your body up into a lunge position. Be careful to keep your abdominal muscles strong as you push your body up. Once you are in a lunge, spring off your back foot, and bring that foot forward next to the other one like you did in the Lunge exercises in Chapter 7.

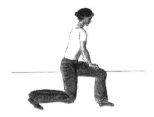

Carry a small backpack instead of a purse

Uneven loads balanced on one shoulder can put undue strain on vertebrae and lead to improper posture. There are many cute backpacks available now that allow you to distribute the weight of your wallet and other purse contents evenly across your back.

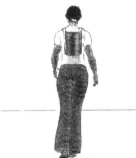

Limit the amount of time you wear high-heeled shoes

High-heels throw your pelvis into a forward tilt and tip your chest back, unnaturally creating too much of an arch in your lower back. Sure they make your calves look sexy, but this position strains the back muscles and vertebrae as your back compensates with extreme curves to keep you balanced.

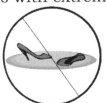

Avoid Bone Robbers

As discussed in Chapter 6, there are many thieves out there preventing your body from properly absorbing vitamins and minerals that are essential for bone strength. Some of theses robbers are diseases. They include rheumatoid arthritis, juvenile diabetes, liver disease, malabsorption diseases, decreased vitamin D metabolism, and reduced stomach acid production. If you are dealing with one of these diseases, you will want to talk to your doctor about taking extra steps to prevent bone loss.

Other robbers that will sabotage your BONES Lifestyle include tobacco, heavy alcohol consumption, medications such as steroids and acid blockers, caffeine, sugars, fats, salt, and processed foods. Dieting to lose weight or following restrictive eating patterns may cause you to leave out necessary vitamins or minerals. It may also cause your body to switch into anti-starvation mode, using stored calcium for life-giving functions such as heart beat and muscle contraction rather than bone density. Stress decreases the absorption of calcium and increases production of adrenal hormones, which stimulate bone loss. And believe it or not, even a lack of sleep is dangerous for your bones. Too little sleep increases stress and the likelihood that you will not follow a proper diet or get enough exercise.

It is unlikely that you will be able to completely eliminate all of the vitamin and mineral robbers from your life, but it is wise to stack the odds in your favor and limit your exposure to them. Live a balanced lifestyle: Make time in your weekly schedule for the BONES Lifestyle exercises; eat the nutritious, colorful foods that are included in the BONES food pyramid; avoid smoking and alcohol; and get plenty of sleep. By taking these simple steps, you will limit the bone robbers' ability to sap your bones' strength.

Congratulations! You're Living the BONES Lifestyle!

So now you understand what osteoporosis is and how it breaks down the bone remodeling system. You've learned that some of the causes of osteoporosis cannot be avoided. You have little control over your genetics, age, illnesses, injuries, or the side effects of prescribed medications.

But you've also seen that these risk factors are only part of the equation. Your lifestyle choices play a major role in maintaining strong bones. If you choose to practice balancing, monitor your bone density with osteoporosis tests, eat nutritious foods, perform bone-building exercises, and take supplements or medication as prescribed by your doctor, then congratulations — you are living the BONES Lifestyle and are on your way to a lifetime of strong, functional bones!

Glossary

androgens

Responsible for development of male sex characteristics. Triggers the bone remodeling cycle in men.

antiresorptive drugs

Medication that stops the resorption (breakdown) of old bone.

bending strength

The ability to resist bending. Requires both tensile strength and compressive strength.

bone density

The amount of bone tissue per cubic centimeter of bones (measured as g/cm3).

bone mass

the amount of bone you have in your body.

bone mineral density (BMD)

The amount of minerals, such as calcium, in a square centimeter of bone. This is measured as g/cm2. An estimate of actual bone density.

bone modeling

The process of bone growth.

bone remodeling

The process of bone growth where additional bone is no longer added, but old, weak, and damaged bone is replaced by new bone.

bone strength

The power of bone to resist force or strain. The resistance to fracture.

center of gravity

The center of your body's weight.

collagen

The most abundant protein in mammals. Long, thin fibrils found in the protein collagen fiber matrix that gives bones flexibility.

compressive force

Force that pushes inward toward the center.

cortical bone

A smooth type of bone tissue, usually found on the outside of bone.

counterbalance

A weight or force that offsets an opposing force.

estrogen

The main sex hormone in women and essential to the menstrual cycle. Also found in men in lower amounts. Affects the bone remodeling cycle.

fatigue fracture
The result of repetitive microdamage typically due to excessive mechanical stress on the bone.

femoral neck
The section of a femur bone that sits just below the ball of the ball–and–socket hip joint and attaches the ball to the long shaft of the femur bone.

formative drugs
Medication that stimulates the osteoblasts and encourages new bone growth.

fragility fracture
A fracture caused by decreased bone strength due to osteoporosis and occurs with very little mechanical stress on the bone.

kyphosis
A curving of the spine that causes a bowing or rounding of the back. Leads to a hunchback or slouching posture.

line of balance
An invisible plumb line that passes through your center of gravity and hangs down from the ceiling, perpendicular to the floor.

lining cells
Pancake–shaped cells that line the outer surface of the bone.

mechanical fatigue
Structural breakdown that occurs when a material is repeatedly loaded and unloaded. Microscopic cracks occur and grow until a fracture occurs.

menopause
The time in a woman's life that her menstruation stops. The ovaries stop making eggs and produce less estrogen and progesterone. Normally occurs between the ages of 45 and 55.

metabolic acidosis
A condition where there is too much acid in body fluids.

neuromuscular system
The interconnectivity of the nervous system, muscular system, and brain. Experienced through the sense of touch — one of the three senses needed for balance.

osteoblasts
Living cells that absorb nutrients from the blood and build new bone.

osteoclasts
Living bone cells that crush old bone and release nutrients into the blood.

osteocytes
Mature osteoblasts that are surrounded by collagen matrix. Sense mechanical strain on the bone.

osteon
The principle organizing feature of cortical bone.

osteopenia
Lower than normal bone mineral density.

osteoporosis
Porous bones.

phytochemicals
Biologically active chemical compounds in plants.

progesterone
A female hormone produced by the ovaries. An important element of the bone remodeling cycle.

tensile force
Force that pulls apart.

testosterone
A male hormone that is responsible for the development of male sexual characteristics. The most potent of the naturally occurring androgens.

trabecular bone
A sponge–like inner structure of bone tissue. Resembles the Eiffel Tower.

vestibular system
Fluid in the middle ear that signals your head's motion to your brain. Related to the sense of hearing — one of the three senses needed for balance.

visual system/vision
Sense of sight. One of the three senses needed for balance.

References

Alexander, R. McNeil. <u>Bones: the Unity of Form and Function</u>. New York: Macmillan, 1994.

Alexander, R. McNeil. <u>Human Bones: a Scientific and Pictorial Investigation</u>. New York: Pl P, an Imprint of Pearson Education, Inc, 2005.

"American Association of Clinical Endocrinologists Medical Guidelines for Clinical Practice for the Prevention and Treatment of Postmenopausal Osteoporosis." <u>Endocrine Practice</u> 9 (2003): 544-564.

Balch, James F., MD, and Phyllis A., CNC Balch. <u>Prescription for Nutritional Healing: a Practical a-Z Reference to Drug-Free Remedies Using Vitamins, Minerals, Herbs & Food Supplements</u>. 2nd ed. Garden City Park, NY: Avery Group, 1997. 413-417.

Bassett, C A. "Fundamental and Practical Aspects of Therapeutic Uses of Pulsed Electromagnetic Fields (PEMFs)." Department of Orthopedic Surgery, Columbia Univ, NY.

Blandine Calais–Germain. <u>Anatomy of Movement</u>. Seattle. Eastland Press, 1993.

Briggs, Andrew M, Greig, Alison M, Wark, John D, Fazzalari, Nicola L, and Bennell, Kim L. "A Review of Anatomical and Mechanical Factors Affecting Vetebral Body Integrity." <u>Int J Med Sci</u>. 2004; 1(3): 170-180.

Bronner, Felix, and Mary C. Farach-Carson. <u>Bone Formation</u>. London: Springer, 2004.

Brown, Susan, E., PhD. <u>Better Bones, Better Body, Beyond Estrogen and Calcium: a Comprehensive Self-Help Program for Preventing, Halting & Overcoming Osteoporosis</u>. New Canaan, Ct: Keats, 2000.

Brown, Susan E., PhD, CCN, and Russell, MD, PhD, CCN Jaffe. "Acid-Alkaline Balance and Its Effect on Bone Health." <u>International Journal of Integrative Medicine</u> 2 (2000).

Burra, Sirisha, et al. "Dendritic Processes of Osteocytes Are Mechanotransducers That Induce the Opening of Hemichannels." <u>Proceedings of the National Academy of Sciences</u>, 2010; DOI: 10.1073/pnas.1009382107.

Comeau, Nicole M. <u>The Relationship Between Calcium, Protein, and Bone Loss in Early Postmenopausal Women</u>. Diss. Oregon State Univ., 2002.

Cowin, Stephen C. <u>Bone Mechanics Handbook</u>. 2nd ed. Boca Raton, FL: CRC P, 2001.

Cowin, Stephen C. <u>Mechanical Properties of Bone</u>, AMD. Vol. 45. New York: The American Society of Mechanical Engineers, 1981.

Currey, John D. <u>Bones: Structure and Mechanics</u>. Princeton and Oxford: Princeton UP, 2002.

Currey, John. The Mechanical Adaptations of Bones. Princeton: Princeton UP, 1984.

Daly, R M., and M A. Petit. "Optimizing Bone Mass and Strength: the Role of Physical Activity and Nutrition During Growth;" Medicine and Sport Science. Vol. 51. Basel Switzerland: Karger, 2007.

Delavier, Frederic. Strength Training Anatomy. 2nd ed. Paris: Human Kinetics, 2006.

"Dietary Protein & Bone Health: New Perspectives." June 2008 <http://www.nationaldairycouncil.org/NationalDairyCouncil/Health/Digest/dcd74-5Page1.htm>.

Evans, F. Gaynor, PhD. Mechanical Properties of Bones. Springfield, Ill: Charles C Thomas Publisher, 1973.

"Fear of falling linked to future falls in older people." BMJ-British Medical Journal (2010, August 22).

Feskanich, D, W C. Willett, and G A. Colditz. "Calcium, Vitamin D, Milk Consumption, and Hip Fractures: a Prospective Study Among Postmenopausal Women." Am J Clin Nutr. 77 (2003): 504-511.

Fong, Kevin. "The Next Small Step." BMJ 329 (2004): 1441-1444.

Fuchs, Robyn K, Cusimano, Barbara, and Snow, Christine M. "Box Jumping: A Bone-Building Exercise for Elementary School Children." JOPERD, Vol. 73, No. 2. Feb. 2002.

Fuchs, Robyn K, Bauer, Jeremy J, and Snow, Christine M. "Jumping Improves Hip and Lumbar Spine Bone Mass in Prepubescent Children: A Randomized Controlled Trial." Journal of Bone and Mineral Research, Vol. 16, No. 1. 2001.

Fullmer, S., PhD, RD, LJ, PhD, RD Moyer-Mileur, DL, PhD Eggett, and AC, PhD Parcell. "Spine and Hip Bone Mineral Density and Current Aerobic Activity in College-Age Women." Journal of the American Dietetic Association 106 (2006): a29. Fall 2007. <http://www.sciencedirect.com/science?_ob=ArticleURL&_udi=B758G-4KG2GYR2P&_user=10&_rdoc=1&_fmt=&_orig=search&_sort=d&view=c&_acct=C000050221&_version=1&_urlVersion=0&_userid=10&md5=443dc20cce1f518d5aaead9a88b9622a>.

Gates, Rhonda, MS, and Beverly, PhD Whipple. Outwitting Osteoporosis. Hillsboro, OR: Beyond Words, 2003.

Gunter, K, Baxter-Jones, ADG, Mirwald, RL, Almstedt, H, Fuchs, RK, Durski, S, Snow, C. "2008 Impact Exercise Increases BMC During Growth: An 8-year Longitudinal Study." Journal of Bone and Mineral Research, 23 (2008): 986-993.

Harry, Jason D, Niemi, James B, Priplata, Attila A, and Collins, James J. "Balancing Act." IEEE Spectrum, pp 36-41. April 2005.

Heaney, Robert P. MD and Barger-Lux, M. Janet. Calcium and Common Sense. New York, Doubleday, 1988.

"Icelandic Company Says It Has Found Osteoporosis Gene." Medical News Today (2003). Summer 2007 <http://www.medicalnewstoday.com/articles/4630.php.>

"II. Osteology, 2. Bone." <u>Grey's Anatomy of the Human Body</u>. 2006 <http://www.bartleby.com/107/18.html>.

Johnell, O, and P Hertzman. "What Evidence is There for the Prevention and Screening of Osteoporosis?" <u>Health Evidence Network Report</u> (2006). May-June 2006 <http://www.euro.who.int/document/e88668.pdf>.

Khan, Karim, Et Al. <u>Physical Activity and Bone Health</u>. Champaign, Ill: Human Kinetics, 2001.

Kraut, Jeffrey A., Delta R. Mishler, Frederick R. Singer, and William G. Goodman. "The Effects of Metabolic Acidosis on Bone Formation and Bone Resorption in the Rat." <u>Kidney International</u> 30 (1986): 694-700.

Littrell, Tonya R. <u>Water Exercise Effects on Bone Density and Fall Risk in Postmenopausal Women</u>. Diss. Oregon State Univ., 2004.

Mayo Clinic. "Treatment Methods are Tailored to the Break." Apr. 1996. <u>Mayo Clinic Health Letter</u>. Vol. 14. 1996. 1-3.

McKay, Heather and Smith, Everett. "Winning the Battle Against Childhood Physical Inactivity: The Key to Bone Strength?" <u>Journal of Bone and Mineral Research</u>, 23 (2008): 980-985.

McNamara, Adrienne J. <u>Bone Mineral Density and Rowing Exercise in Older Women</u>. Diss. Oregon State Univ., 2005. 2005.

Meeks, Sara, PT, GCS. <u>Walk Tall! an Exercise Program for the Prevention and Treatment of Osteoporosis</u>. Gainesville, FL: Triad, 1999.

Midura, R J., M O. Ibiwoye, K A. Powell, Y Sakai, T Doehring, M D. Grabiner, T E. Patterson, M Zborowski, and A Wolfman. "Pulsed Electromagnetic Field Treatments Enhance the Healing of Fibular Osteotomies." <u>J Orthop Res</u> 5 (2005): 1035-1046.

"Minerals." Linus Pauling Institute. Micronutrient Information Center. Spring 2008 <http://lpi.oregonstate.edu/infocenter/minerals.html>.

Muhlbauer, R.C., Et Al. "Effect of Vegetables on Bone Metabolism." <u>Nature</u> 401 (1999): 343-344.

Muhlbauer, RC, F Li, A Lozano, A Reinli, T Tschudi, and Bone Biology Group, Dept . "Some Vegetables (Commonly Consumed by Humans) Efficiently Modulate Bone Metabolism." <u>J Musculoskel Neuron Interact</u> 1 (2000): 137-140.

Nachemson, Alf. "The Lumbar Spine: An Orthopaedic Challenge." <u>Spine</u>, Vol. 1, No. 1. March 1976.

Nachemson, Alf. "Towards a Better Understanding of Low-Back Pain: A Review of the Mechanics of the Lumbar Disc." <u>Rheumatology and Rehabilitation</u>, Vol. XIV No. 3. 14, 129-143. 1975.

National Osteoporosis Foundation (NOF). <http://www.nof.org/>.

Nestle, Marion. <u>Food Politics</u>. Berkeley: University of California P, 2002.

New, S A., S P. Robins, M K. Campbell, J C. Martin, C Bolton-Smith, D A. Grubb, S J. Lee, and D M. Reid. "Dietary Influences on Bone Mass and Bone Metabolism: Further Evidence of a Positive Link Between Fruit and Vegetable Consumption and Bone Health?" <u>American Journal of Clinical Nutrition</u> 71 (2000): 142-151.

Newman, Renee. <u>Osteoporosis Prevention</u>. Los Angeles, CA. International Jewelry Publications, Inc., 2006.

Notelovitz, Morris, MD, PhD. <u>Stand Tall: Every Woman's Guide to Preventing and Treating Osteoporosis</u>. 2nd ed. Gainesville, FL: Triad Company, 1998.

O'Connor, Carolyn Riester, MD, and Sharon, RN Perkins. <u>Osteoporosis for Dummies</u>. Indianapolis, Indiana: Wiley, Inc., 2005.

Peck, William A. <u>Bone and Mineral Research</u>. Vol. 6. Amsterdam: Elsevier Science, 1989.

"Phytochemicals." Linus Pauling Institute. Micronutrient Information Center. Spring 2008 <http://lpi.oregonstate.edu/infocenter/phytochemicals.html>.

Putnam, SE, AM Scutt, K Bicknell, CM Priestly, and EM Williamson. "Natural Products as Alternative Treatments for Metabolic Bone Disorders and for Maintenance of Bone Health." <u>Phytother Res</u>, School of Pharmacy, University of Reading 21 (2007): 99-112.

Qing Zhang, Esteban Cuartas, Nozer Mehta, James Gilligan, Hua-Zhu Ke, W. Mark Saltzman, Maya Kotas, Mandy Ma, Sonali Rajan, Cecile Chalouni, Jodi Carlson, Agnes Vignery. "Replacement of Bone Marrow by Bone in Rat Femurs: The Bone Bioreactor." <u>Tissue Engineering</u>, 14 (2). 2008. doi:10.1089/ten.2007.0261.

Robling AG, Hinant FM, Burr DB, Turner CH. "Improved Bone Structure and Strength After Long-term Mechanical Loading is Greatest if Loading is Separated Into Short Bouts." <u>Journal of Bone and Mineral Research: The Official Journal of the American Society for Bone and Mineral Research (J Bone Miner Res)</u>. Vol. 17 (8), pp 1545-54. 2002.

Rohr, Christine I., Arup Sarkar, Kimberly R., PhD Barber, and John M., MPA Clements. "Prevalence of Prevention and Treatment Modalities Used in Population At Risk of Osteoporosis." <u>Journal of the American Osteopathic Association</u> 10 (2004): 281-286.

Roy J, MD, PhD, DPE. <u>Aging, Physical Activity, and Health</u>. Champaign, Ill: Human Kinetics, 1997.

Rubin, Clinton, Recker, Robert, Cullen, Diane, Ryaby, John, McCabe, Joan, and McLeodShephard. Kenneth. "Prevention of Postmenopausal Bone Loss by a Low-Magnitude, High-Frequency Mechanical Stimuli: A Clinical Trial Assessing Compliance Efficacy, and Safety," <u>Journal of Bone and Mineral Research</u>. 19(3), 2004. doi: 10.1359/JBMR.0301251.

Shaw, Janet M and Snow, Christine. "Osteoporosis and Physical Activity." <u>PCPFS Research Digest</u>, Series 2, No. 3.

Shaw, Janet M and Snow, Christine. "Weighted Vest Exercise Improves Indices of Fall Risk in Older Women." Journal of Gerontology: Medical Sciences, Vol. 53, No. 1, M53-M58. 1998.

Snow, Christine, PhD. "Exercise Prescription: Building Back Strength." The Osteoporosis Report. National Osteoporosis Foundation. 2003.

Snow, Christine M, Shaw, Janet M, Winters, Kerri M, and Witzke, Kara A. "Long-term Exercise Using Weighted Vests Prevents Hip Bone Loss in Postmenopausal Women." Journal of Gerontology: Medical Sciences, Vol. 55A, No. 9, M489-M491. 2000.

Snowden, D.A., Et Al. "Antioxidents and Reduced Functional Capacity in the Elderly: Findings From the Nun Study." Journal of Gerontology: Medical Sciences 51A (1966): m10-m16.

Tsiaras, Alexander, and Werth Barry. The Architecture and Design of Man and Woman. New York: Doubleday, 2004.

Turner, Charles H. "The biomechanics of hip fracture." The Lancet (July 9, 2005). Vol. 366 No. 9480 pp 98-99

University of Texas Health Science Center at San Antonio (2010, July 20). "Bone Cells' Branches Sense Stimulation, When To Make New Bone." ScienceDaily. Retrieved July 21, 2010, from http://www.sciencedaily.com/releases/2010/07/100720123637.htm.

"USDA National Nutrient Database for Standard Reference." USDA Nutrient Data Laboratory (2008). Spring 2008 <http://www.nal.usda.gov/fnic/foodcomp/search/>.

"Vitamins." Linus Pauling Institute. Micronutrient Information Center. Spring 2008 <http://lpi.oregonstate.edu/infocenter/vitamins.html>.

White, Martha. Cotler H.B. The Aging Spine: Water Exercise and Treatment Principles. New York: iUniverse, 2004.

Wiley, John & Sons, Ltd. "Phytochemicals." PubMed (2006).

Winters, Kerri M and Snow, Christine M. "Detraining Reverses Positive Effects of Exercise on the Musculoskeletal System in Premenopausal Women." Journal of Bone and Mineral Research, Vol. 15, No. 12. 2000.

Index

G

genetic test 193–194
golden threesome 34–36
  sight 26–27, 34–35
  sound 26–27, 34–35
  touch 26–27, 34–35

H

hip 18, 21-24
hormone replacement therapies (ERT or HRT) 182-183, 186
humerus 4–5

J

jump 109–110, 142-143

K

kyphosis 39, 60

L

line of balance 36–42
lining cells 9–12

M

magnesium 29, 83, 85
manganese 87
mechanical fatigue 110, 114
menopause 19–21
minerals 4–12
modeling 14–16
modifications 148
muscle mass 60
muscle memory 105

N

National Osteoporosis Foundation (NOF) 21, 61
neutral pelvis 119

O

occipital joint 39
osteoblasts 9–12, 14–18
osteoclasts 8–12, 14–18
osteocytes 9–12
osteon 2, 11
osteopenia 11, 17, 20
osteoporosis 11, 17, 20

P

peak bone mineral density 14, 112
pelvic girdle 119
pelvis 40–41
periodontal disease 60
peripheral dual–energy x–ray absorptiometry (PDXA)
  62, 65
peripheral quantitative computed tomography (pQCT)
  62, 65
peripheral tests 63
phosphorus 86
pH scale 94–95
phytochemicals 93–94
posture 36–51
potassium 83, 86
progesterone 19
protein 91

Q

quantitative ultrasonography (QUS) 62, 65

R

radiographic absorptiometry (RA) 62, 64
remodeling 16–18, 182
risk factors for osteoporosis 58–59
roll-drop-lock 120
  modified roll-drop-lock 152
rules of engagement 119

S

sacral arrow 40–41
sacrum 40
safety precautions 117
selective estrogen receptor modulators (SERMS) 183,
  187
severe osteoporosis 75, 148
shoulder girdle 119
silica 87
single energy x–ray absorptiometry (SXA) 62, 64
site-directed bone growth (SDBG) 190–191
sodium flouride 183, 185
sulfur 88

T

tendon 31
tensile force 6
teriparatide 183, 185

testerone 19
thoracic breathing 46–47
tibia 4–5
tissue regeneration 189–190
trabecular bone 2, 16–17
tripod of the foot 41
T-score 66–69

U

United States Department of Agriculture (USDA) 78

V

vertebra, vertebrae 18, 21–23, 39–41
  cervical vertebra 39
  lumbar vertebra 40
  thoracic vertebra 39–40, 46–47
vibration therapy 191–192
vitamin A 88, 181
vitamin B5 89
vitamin B6 89
vitamin B9 89
vitamin B12 29, 90
vitamin C 90
vitamin D 29, 83, 90, 181
vitamin E 90
vitamin K 29, 91

W

wrist 18, 21–23

Z

zinc 29, 88
Z-score 69

Made in the USA
San Bernardino, CA
25 May 2016